STATE MENTAL HOSPITALS

STATE MENTAL HOSPITALS
Problems and Potentials

Edited by

John A. Talbott, M.D.

Cornell University Medical College
New York, New York

The Payne-Whitney Psychiatric Clinic
The New York Hospital
New York, New York

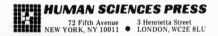 **HUMAN SCIENCES PRESS**

72 Fifth Avenue   3 Henrietta Street
NEW YORK, NY 10011 ● LONDON, WC2E 8LU

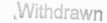

90074

Copyright © 1980 by Human Sciences Press, Inc.
72 Fifth Avenue, New York, New York 10011

Printed in the United States of America
0123456789 987654321

Library of Congress Cataloging in Publication Data

Main Entry under title:

State mental hospitals

   1. Psychiatric hospitals—United States.
2. Hospitals, State—United States. I. Talbott,
John A. [DNLM: 1. Hospitals, Psychiatric—United
States. 2. Hospitals, Public—United States.
WM27 AA1 S77]
RC443.S83   362.2'1'0973   LC 79-21928
ISBN 0-87705-394-4

CONTENTS

ACKNOWLEDGMENTS

It is with deep appreciation that I acknowledge the contributions of Leon Salzman, M.D., and Lawrence C. Kolb, M.D., to this enterprise. It was Dr. Salzman, a member of the program committee of the American Psychiatric Association, who first suggested to me that it would be fruitful to take a fresh look at the problem of state hospitals. And it was Dr. Kolb, then Commissioner of Mental Hygiene in New York State, who after listening to the first special section on the topic, at the APA Annual Meeting, suggested that there was adequate material for a book on the subject. To Drs. Salzman and Kolb, to all the contributers and their staffs, and especially to *my* past and present staffs—my deepest gratitude.

CONTRIBUTORS

A. ANTHONY ARCE, M.D. is Director, Hahnemann Community Mental Health and Retardation Center and Professor of Psychiatry, Hahnemann Medical College and Hospital of Philadelphia.

JAMES BARTER, M.D. is Director of Residency Training, Department of Psychiatry, University of California-Davis Medical Center, Division of Mental Health, Sacramento California.

HENRY BRILL M.D. is former Deputy Commissioner, New York State Department of Mental Hygiene and Clinical Professor of Psychiatry, State University of New York at Stonybrook.

ROBERT M. DALY, M.D. is Chairman, Department of Psychiatry, Park City Hospital, Bridgeport, Connecticut and Director of In-Patient Services, Park City Hospital.

ROBERT DEVITO, M.D. is Director of the Department of Mental Health and Developmental Disabilities for the State of Illinois.

JACK EWALT, M.D. is Director of Mental Health and Behavioral Science Service, Veterans Administration, Washington, D.C.

RICHARD N. FILER, PH.D. is former Deputy Assistant Chief Medical Director for Extended Care, Veterans Administration, Washington, D.C.

IRWIN M. GREENBERG, M.D., D.M.S.C. is Director of Psychiatric Services, Waterbury Hospital Health Center and Associate Clinical Professor of Psychiatry, Yale University School of Medicine.

J. FRANK JAMES, M.D. is Director of the State Department of Mental Health, State of Oklahoma.

STUART L. KEILL, M.D. is Chairman of the Department of Psychiatry and Psychology and Professor of Clinical Psychiatry, State University of New York at Stonybrook.

LAWRENCE C. KOLB, M.D. is Distinguished Physician in Psychiatry, Veterans Administration Hospital, Albany, New York and Professor Emeritus of Psychiatry, Columbia University College of Physicians and Surgeons.

LEE B. MACHT, M.D. is Professor and Chairman, Department of Psychiatry, Harvard Medical School at the Cambridge Hospital and Chief, Department of Psychiatry at the Cambridge Hospital.

JOHN A. TALBOTT, M.D. is Professor of Psychiatry, Cornell University Medical College and Associate Medical Director, Payne Whitney Clinic—-The New York Hospital.

FRANCIS A. TYCE, M.D. is Medical Director and Chief Executive Officer, Rochester State Hospital, Rochester, Minnesota.

ISRAEL ZWERLING, M.D., PH.D. is Professor and Chairman, Department of Mental Health Sciences, Hahnemann Medical College and Hospital of Philadelphia.

FOREWORD

Lawrence C. Kolb, M.D.

For the vast majority of those in our nation, the state hospitals for the care of the mentally ill and retarded are unknown or perceived as frightening or irresponsible institutions. They stimulate thoughts of hopelessness as the final destination of men and women so demented or socially threatening that confinement is their proper due. Also, their staffs are accused of irresponsibility as a few of their former patients now are recognized on the streets as a consequence of their bizarre or socially distressing behavior or dramatically reported in the news for some act of violence.

These general misperceptions of the seriously mentally ill are ingrained stereotypes held by many—stereotypes that, in fact, led to the development of the state, county, and federal hospital systems to care for the socially impaired mentally disabled. These attitudes were responsible for the isolation of the institutions from communities; they were pervasive over the years in decision-making as regards provision of tax monies for their support. Today such attitudes continue to delay and distort the vast and humane forward move in the care of the mentally disabled.

Contrary to these perniciously held stereotypes of the state hospitals, such facilities have been in the vortex of vast change during the past several decades. That change probably derived more from technological advance in the field of psychiatry— through the introduction of highly effective psychophar- maceuticals that have radically altered the extent and degree of psychotic abnormal behavior—than from other important forces. These other forces are the more open and accepting attitudes of the general public towards the mentally ill, those sociological studies that examined the social structures of men- tal hospitals, postulated the deleterious effect of prolonged insti- tutional care in the closed institutional milieu, and delineated the "social breakdown syndrome" as a secondary consequence of such care. Britain's open hospital movement preceded and stimulated the community mental health movement sponsored by this nation's federal government. So did the various experi- ences in Europe of a variety of alternative approaches to the care of the mentally ill, including the day hospitals and psy- choneurological dispensary care of the USSR.

Two decades ago, the dramatic statement of Dr. Harry Solomon made during his Presidential Address for the Ameri- can Psychiatric Association calling for the closure of the state hospitals represented an attack upon the state hospital system as a symbol of a type of insensitive, depersonalized, and immov- able bureautically administered system. That statement then probably provoked and angered more of his professional col- leagues than it pleased. At the time the state systems provided the bulk of mental health care throughout the country. Few discerned that the turn of events had already occurred when Dr. Solomon uttered these words, that the decline of the state hospital care system was already underway. That change has proceeded apace throughout the world, as alternative psychiat- ric facilities have sprung up in general hospital systems, the federal community mental health centers, and as communities have offered other residential and rehabilitative centers. But there have emerged as well glaring examples of the limitations of the narrow applications of both the psychopharmaceutical and sociological resolutions to caring for these impaired mentally ill with serious and persistent personality deficits. As the residents of all communities will attest, there remains a nucleus of individuals discharged thereto whose psychotic impairments disclose their imperviousness to both modern medical prescription and societal stimulation. These individuals form the hardcore groups of schizophrenics and brain-damaged persons in whom the capacity for social adaptation is limited due to the unmodifiable nature of their personality disorder or the irreversibility of brain damage. These are the persons who have been cared for and hidden over the last century within the state hospitals—these as well as many others whose recoveries are expedited today by the modern therapeutic approaches. These chronically impaired individuals must be recognized as existing by administrators, program planners, and therapists within the general and mental health system. The planners and administrators must provide and continue to provide for them humane and interested caretakers and appropriate facilities. The delusion must be dispelled that modern biopsychosocial therapies have done away with chronicity of socially impairing behavior in many who have and will suffer psychoses.

The editor of *State Mental Hospitals* has brought together an extraordinary group of contributors as writers of various chapters in this book. Physicians all, they have elected a most challenging task in modern psychiatry—the administration of the modern state hospital or the administration of therapeutic programs affiliated or linked to such. One is now a commissioner of a state hospital program. Beyond that, and as this commentator personally has observed, they have demonstrated in their leadership roles the capacity to face the crises and adversities inherent in operation of institutions caring for the most behaviorally disturbed. They have brought innovative leadership and worked with thoughtful appreciation of the many forces now radically altering the state hospital delivery system.

In Part I of this volume, the descriptions of the recent problems of the state hospitals represent a distillate of personal experience given by this highly sensitive and perceptive group of psychiatric administrators. They have responded in their writing with an impressive and engaging analytic perspicacity, humor, indignation, and creative suggestions.

In Part II, the reader will find a variety of suggestions as to the future potentials for operation of state hospitals; they range from consideration of their complete closure to a variety of alternatives, some already in test, as integral units in the totality of the mental health system. There is no doubt a continuing need in the mental health system for a facility of some kind in place and functioning to provide continuous and compassionate care to those with chronically impairing disabilities. Recent experience has demonstrated the necessity that the housing of such services be so arranged that those served neither unduly distress the local community nor be exposed, as some are today, to the neglect or abuse of a nonaccepting ingroup of community residents.

Those concerned with the future role of the state hospital and the mental health delivery system will be engaged, saddened, stimulated, and amused by these essays. They may well wish a further elaboration of the incapacity of our policy planners and political leaders to solve the existing and inevitable difficulties of the problem of direct delivery of mental health services by perpetuations of the discontinuities inherent in services provided simultaneously by three levels of government, as well as competing, voluntary and proprietary systems. This commentator patiently continues to wait for courageous and nonaligned political and professional leaders to group and untangle the knots that have so strongly been tied by ill thought through political, legislative, administrative, and regulatory efforts. Perhaps, like the fisherman confronted by his tangled line, the solution rests in several well defined cuts—with substitution of a single string and new line—even though initially costly.

PREFACE

The future of state mental hospitals is or should be of major concern to all persons in the field of mental health. State hospitals have been criticized for their inhumane conditions, inadequate treatment programs and incompetent if not brutal staffs since their growth mushroomed in the mid-19th century.

Newer facilities, such as psychopathic hospitals, general hospital psychiatric units, Veterans Administration hospitals and community mental health centers were established in the 20th century to treat the severely mentally ill. However, state hospitals continued, as before, relatively unaffected by these developments, although they currently are in a declining phase.

Deinstitutionalization is the newest development affecting state hospitals and has been characterized by an unplanned but intentional movement of the severely and chronically mentally ill from state facilities to community settings. It is immaterial now, whether the motives behind deinstitutionalization were philosophical (e.g. the community mental health movement), therapeutic (e.g. advances in technology, especially psycho-

pharmacology), or economic (e.g. shifting the burden for pay-
ment of care of the mentally ill from state-supported mental
hospitals to federally-funded nursing homes and welfare ho-
tels). Deinstitutionalization, by reducing the census both nationwide and in individual hospitals, has left the state facility
in limbo, no longer either custodial asylum and institution of
last resort for society's mental rejects, nor active, community-
related and quality-oriented service, able to care for the very
population it was designed to serve—the severely and chronically mentally ill. In addition, the entire mental health system,
or non-system, as the case may be, is also in limbo, unable to
utilize the resources of the state facility to care for this population, either in hospital or in community settings. Although the
census in the state hospitals has declined to one-third its former
high, the monies previously allocated to care for the no-longer
institutionalized two-thirds are not available to local community services to care for the almost massive number of deinstitutionalized patients.

Bearing in mind that both state hospitals and the mental
health system find themselves in this state of limbo, this volume
examines the problems encountered by state hospitals and proposes practical and urgently needed solutions to these problems.

PREVIEW

Part I, the Introduction, presents an overview of the problems encountered by state mental hospitals. From these problems, several solutions suggest themselves, most prominent
among them an alteration of the role of the state facility.

In Part II, several authors provide detailed descriptions of
the specific problems of state hospitals. Irwin Greenberg places
their problems in historical perspective in Chapter 2; A. Anthony Arce describes the governmental influences and stric-
tures prevalent in Chapter 3; Israel Zwerling provides details of

both the problems and promise of university affiliations in Chapter 4; Stuart Keill and the editor provide two linked summaries of the manpower problems and role of professionals as well as characteristics of state hospital leaders in Chapters 5 and 6; and Robert Daly concludes this part with a case description of the demise of vitality of a state hospital in Chapter 7.

Part III deals with the potential role and probable future of the state hospital. In Chapter 8, Frank James suggests that state hospitals will and should be replaced; in Chapter 9, Henry Brill argues that they should be retained until something better is found; in Chapter 10, James Barter writes of the need for state hospitals to perform specialized or tertiary functions; in Chapter 11, Richard Filer and Jack Ewalt argue that the Veterans Hospital experience with domiciliary care facilities may pertain to the new role of the state facility; and in Chapter 12, Frank Tyce suggests most emphatically that state hospitals, despite their limitations, can successfully function as comprehensive community mental health services.

The conclusion of the book, Part IV, consists of two presentations by Robert De Vito and Lee Macht, both of whom have occupied commissionerships in recent years, during trying times. Using their experience, they give guidelines for the future of both the state hospital and state psychiatric services.

John A. Talbott, M.D.

Part I

INTRODUCTION

Chapter 1

THE PROBLEMS AND POTENTIAL ROLES OF THE STATE MENTAL HOSPITAL

John A. Talbott, M.D.

The literature on the problems of state hospitals is extensive but not particularly helpful. The two best known and most effective critiques of mental hospitals in this century were written, not by mental health professionals, but by interested, involved, concerned citizens. Clifford Beers's book, *A Mind That Found Itself,*[1] while not written about a state mental hospital, highlighted the inhumane conditions, callous staff attitudes, and lack of effective treatment and care prevalent in mental hospitals at the turn of the century. Later, Albert Deutsch's *Shame of the States*[2] further documented the overcrowding, horrid conditions, and seemingly barbaric practices prevalent in state mental hospitals nationwide.

One of the primary purposes of the Joint Commission on Mental Health and Illness (1955-60) was to address the problem of the state hospital, and its summary report, *Action for Mental Health,*[3] called for a halt in construction of new state hospitals containing over 1,000 beds, the conversion of existing state hospitals into facilities for the chronically medically ill, and the establishment of a network of community mental health clinics. The federal legislation resulting from this report, heralded by President John F. Kennedy's call for a "bold new approach"[4] was intended in large part to decrease our dependence on state hospitals through the use of community mental health centers.

In 1975, Zusman and Bertsch published *The Future Role of the State Hospital,*[5] which while indicating the state of thinking at that time, led to no firm conclusions as to directions for state mental hospitals. Most recently, Leona Bachrach summarized the literature in her study on deinstitutionalization,[6] which again highlighted the problems of both institutional and deinstitutional care but produced no firm conclusions as to future direction.

THE PROBLEMS OF STATE HOSPITALS

The problems encountered by state mental hospitals can be grouped into 11 areas. These are: physical plants; patients; staff; treatment programs; service systems; state mental health departments; other state departments and agencies; state legislatures; outside agencies and forces; lack of a constituency; and lack of funding.

1. *Physical Plants.* State hospital buildings frequently pose insuperable problems. Most buildings are old or were constructed using outdated architectural plans or ideas; are located far from the urban areas they serve; are inflexible in their architectural design; are drab and "institutional"; stress safety and structure rather than programs and function; and utilize dormitory housing rather than single or double rooms, which afford more privacy. Naturally there are exceptions, most notably the newer zone centers in Illinois and quasi-community mental health centers in New York State, but the majority suffer from antiquated plants.

2. *Patients.* The patients served in state hospitals represent a public health responsibility for the facility. Until the last decade, no one was denied service who needed it, and persons deemed suitable for admission by the community were admitted without question. Because of this public health responsibility, the patients admitted to state hospitals tend to be readmissions rather than first-admissions; they tend to be schizophrenic or organic rather than manic-depressive or characterological; they tend to be chronic rather than acute; and they tend to cluster in the lower socioeconomic groups. In short, they are the patients for whom the state facility is the hospital of last resort. Again, there are exceptions: state facilities are reaching out with greater effectiveness into the community with aftercare and outpatient treatment of the never-hospitalized; they offer treatment of abusers of drugs or alcohol; and they provide emergency and crisis intervention services.

3. *Staff.* The staff serving in state facilities is also part of the problem. The staff tends to reflect the low status and civil service mentality prevalent in state service; they are often (especially in urban areas) of the same low socioeconomic status as the patients; they are frequently less educated and less well-trained than their counterparts in community hospitals; they frequently see patient care as a job like any other civil service job, that is, in terms of security, rights, and pensions; and among physicians there is a higher percentage of foreign medical graduates (FMG's) whose language and cultural differences may pose significant problems.

4. *Treatment Programs.* While most state hospitals have abandoned purely custodial care and initiated more active treatment and rehabilitation, there is still a reliance on drugs and quasi-therapeutic milieus, e.g. group treatment, therapeutic communities and patient government, as opposed to full day involvement in active psychotherapy, socialization, and rehabilitation activities. There is also, by necessity, an emphasis

on quantity, not quality; on holding actions rather than progress; and on nonmedical interventions.

5. *Service Systems.* Since the state hospital is part of a larger mental health system, it shares the problems of the larger system. These include: the fragmentation and lack of coordination between elements in the system; a conflict of interest inherent when all levels of government both run their own services and contract with others to run them; and the bewildering multiplicity of governmental funding and administration—e.g., federally funded VA hospitals and Community Mental Health Centers, state funded state hospitals, city and county funded hospitals, and voluntary hospitals and clinics. Again, there are exceptions to absolute fragmentation in such states as Arizona, which has attempted to coordinate administration of all services, and New York State, which has attempted a "unified services" approach; but these efforts remain isolated and incomplete.

6. *State Departments of Mental Health.* State departments of mental health, at least in the larger states, pose additional problems for the state facilities. State departments tend to think in terms of centralized functions rather than decentralization; they tend to emphasize bureaucratic needs over patient care; tend to stress cost containment rather than quality of care; they tend to work to maintain themselves rather than encourage locally developed competence and services; and often they are politically unsophisticated.

7. *Other Departments or Agencies in the State Government.* Agencies such as Civil Service, Budget, Audit and Control, Health, and Social Services pose additional problems for the state hospital. Preoccupied as they usually are with the promulgation of regulations, inspections, paperwork, turf, and competition for scarce resources, it is no wonder that they are seen almost solely as harassing bodies rather than collaborative, cooperative, or facilitating agencies. In addition, their dominance by professional civil servants, lawyers, and accountants

further widens their distance from patients and mental health professionals.

8. *State Legislatures.* Dependent as they are on state coffers for operating expenses and programs, state hospitals are literally at the mercy of state legislators. Given their lack of a constituency and the stigma of serious mental illness, it is not surprising that state hospitals are underfunded, undercared for, and misunderstood. Despite the fact that mental health constitutes the highest, or second highest, area of expenditure for a state, legislators tend to be concerned only with scandals in the state hospital system rather than with developing an ongoing concern with the perpetual problems inherent in the system; and they use state hospital conditions only during election campaigns—the party in power manipulating the attrition and hiring patterns, the opposition party attacking the care and scandalous conditions present in the facilities.

9. *Outside Agencies or Forces.* To add to the state hospitals' already overwhelming list of problems, the proliferation of outside agencies and forces in recent years has made them almost beleaguered institutions. For instance, in addition to the accrediting bodies, most central of them being the Joint Commission on the Accreditation of Hospitals, there are now 156 agencies that have authority to monitor and inspect hospitals in New York State. Add to these the growing number of judicial actions, patients rights groups, citizens groups, and media investigations, and some insight into the pressure felt by state hospitals may be gained.

10. *The Lack of a Constituency.* A major problem of state hospitals is the lack of an informed, concerned, and vocal constituency to lobby and fight for monies, programs, and services. Mental patients probably fare the worst of all groups underserved and discriminated against. Even welfare mothers and prisoners enjoy stronger advocacy efforts. And within the mental health field, advocates for the chronic mental patient are few in comparison with those concerned with the mentally re-

tarded, the alcoholic, or the drug addict. With few intact family members, still fewer friends, and no political contacts, it is no wonder their voice is small.

11. *Lack of Adequate Funding.* State hospitals, in large part because of their patient population, physical plants, lack of a constituency, low status, stigma of chronic mental illness, and lack of legislative support, have traditionally been inadequately funded. This, plus the pressure to avoid scandal, keep disturbed persons off the streets, and serve the rest of the mental health system's rejects and failures, make for an overwhelming problem.

What Changes Are Needed

To change the situation in state hospitals for the better and improve the lot of the severely and chronically mentally ill population they are mandated to serve, several areas need to be addressed. These are: societal and professional attitudes, funding priorities and mechanisms, administrative structures and procedures, and program planning and implementation.

Societal and professional attitudes toward the chronically mentally ill and state mental hospitals are critical to any substantive change. As long as both are accorded low status, differential funding, and maximal stigmatization, there is slim hope for improvement. A broad-based attack on existing public attitudes must be initiated to inform the public about the price it is paying for a fragmented, second-rate system of care for its most needy. Medicine, psychiatry, and all mental health professions must also alter their educational curricula, the role models they offer in training programs, and their placements for training experiences.

Funding priorities and mechanisms are in need of a similar attack. Funding priorities must be altered to address the most critical problems first, relegating to a minor status less severe problems. Funding mechanisms must be altered drastically so that federal support is no longer fragmented but directed at real recipients; so that states are able to shift resources from state facilities to local services; and so that patients have some choice in selecting effective local treatment and care, such as a voucher system would provide.

Administrative structures and procedures must be revised. Governments should be divested of the conflict of interest situation of both managing and contracting for mental health services. Duplication in the governmental layers must be eliminated. Currently, everyone wants to plan, monitor, and promulgate regulations, but no one seems interested in improving the quality of care for patients. There must be an eventual shift toward a flow of monies and responsibility from federal to state to local services, so that broad policy is set at the top and programs and treatment are implemented at the base.

Program planning and implementation must also be addressed. Clear goals and objectives must be formulated, articulated, and implemented. No longer should state hospitals and chronic mental patients be given short shrift and then blamed for their shortcomings. In addition, a unified approach must be adopted so that there can be an end to the city-state-federal struggles for shifting funding burdens, grabbing or abandoning turf, and assessing blame. Clear roles must be defined for all participants in the mental health system.

THE POTENTIAL ROLES OF STATE HOSPITALS

There are four generally accepted options for state hospitals given the problems outlined above: closure, maintenance of the status quo, radical reform, and alterations in function. Efforts to effect closure seem to have stalled across the nation; in light of the backlash to deinstitutionalization without adequate community supports and community services, closure no longer seems an immediate possibility. Efforts to retain state hospitals as they currently exist seem increasingly unlikely, given the continuing difficulties experienced by the facilities, the barrage of criticism directed toward them, and the renewed interest in the treatment and care of the chronic mental patient. Radical reform of all the offending elements involved in creating the disasters present in the state hospital system—e.g., civil service, bureaucratic insensitivity, poor funding, low status, etc.—also seems too idealistic for current times. Therefore, alteration in functioning seems to be the easiest, most likely, and most feasible option open to the state hospital. Such a solution would not endanger jobs, threaten local businesses, or eliminate entrenched bureaucracies. Instead, it would retain the existing buildings, staff, and administrative structures, while altering the task performed.

Several roles have been suggested for the state facility in the future: that of community mental health center, tertiary care facility, domiciliary care facility, and multipurpose mental health service that would accommodate the gaps in service as part of a comprehensive, unified network of services.

It is impossible to predict which of these options will be the one taken by the shapers of policy for the state system. But one or more must prevail, because the system is tottering on the brink of disaster—financially and clinically—and some change is inevitable.

REFERENCES

1. Beers C.: *A Mind That Found Itself.* Garden City, N. Y.: Doubleday, 1908.

2. Deutsch, A.: *Shame of the States.* Garden City, N. Y.: Doubleday, 1937.

3. Joint Commission on Mental Health and Illness: *Action for Mental Health.* New York: Basic Books, 1961.

4. Kennedy, J. F.: "Message from the President of the United States relative to mental illness and mental retardation" *American Journal of Psychiatry* 120: 729–737, 1964.

5. Zusman, B. & Bertsch, E. F.: *The Future Role of the State Hospital.* Lexington, Mass.: Lexington Press, 1975.

6. Bachrach, L. L.: Deinstitutionalization: An analytical review and sociological perspective. Rockville, Md.: National Institute of Mental Health, 1976.

Part II

THE PROBLEMS OF STATE HOSPITALS

Chapter 2

SOCIAL CALVINSIM, FREE WILL, ETIOLOGY, AND TREATMENT

Irwin M. Greenberg, M.D., D.M.SC.

INTRODUCTION

Institutions, whether constructed of matter in the physical world, or of ideas and attitudes in the social world, do not arise or decline *de novo*. Most often, they develop to fulfill a perceived need, either of a critical number of members of a society, or of a smaller but more powerful group.[1] When the need is no longer perceived, the institution declines or changes. It is therefore not surprising that the state mental hospital, an institution with both material and ideological components, has undergone such a progression, with a sharp rise during the late nineteenth and early twentieth centuries, and a fairly rapid alteration, if not decline, in the second half of the twentieth century. The purpose of this discussion is to outline some of the social, ideological, and scientific forces that appear to have contributed to this process, and to raise some questions concerning the care of persons with psychiatric illness, particularly severe illness, in the future. There is a covert axiom here, which, when stated explicitly, asserts (1) that there does indeed exist real psychiatric illness and (2) that while some behavioral reaction patterns that are termed "illness" may indeed be determined by social conditions, these are *not* the illnesses addressed here.

The most powerful social force contributing to the birth of the state hospital system was probably the classical Industrial Revolution, which reached its zenith at about the same time that state hospitals became recognizable institutions, and formed the social system known as the state hospital system.[2,3] The ideological forces were those of Social Darwinism and Social Calvinism, and the relevant scientific forces lay in the areas of profound advances in tissue pathology and the etiology of infectious diseases. The forces that maintained the system were in general, the same, but with some specific differences, e.g., the decline of the extended family, urbanization, and anomie.[4] It is these same forces that currently encourage the maintenance as well as the decline or alteration of the system. There are, however, newer events and ideas that have contributed— and are still contributing—to the decline or change in state hospitals. The newer social forces consist of the society's progression to what has been termed "postindustrial" or "affluent society," the rise of the middle classes and changes in demographic patterns. Ideologically, the new avowed values of many of the world's societies indicate that many of the principles of Social Darwinism and Social Calvinism are no longer acceptable, and are being replaced by a more universal egalitarianism. Lastly, the new scientific advances in technology and medicine have led to the prolongation of life as well as to the capability of saving many lives at birth, thus giving rise to several biologically, but not genetically, impaired populations with psychiatric *symptoms* as part of other biologically determined illnesses. Moreover, the treatment armamentarium of psychiatry has expanded to an almost unbelievable degree.

These forces will be discussed both separately and with respect to their interactions.

THE INDUSTRIAL REVOLUTION

It is clearly not the purpose of this discussion to define or elaborate on the Industrial Revolution. What appears to be of greatest significance are the direct effects on the masses of people involved in terms of the development of recognizable psychiatric illness as well as the indirect effects of the treatment methods developed for those illnesses. Many people displaced themselves to foreign countries, from farm to city, and from family to social anomie of larger cities, as a result of their search for factory employment. Without taking great liberties, it may be surmised that some of those people suffered from biological predisposition to illness, such as in the schizphrenias and the major affective disorders, and that others were subject to metabolic and infectious disorders (e.g., lues) with primary or secondary psychiatric symtoms.[2] Given the lack of social and familial support in newly industrialized society, it might be safe to assume that the interaction of biological and psychosocial disorder produced large numbers of people with structured psychiatric symptoms, particularly within the immigrant populations and their children in the urbanized centers.[5]

The understanding of the etiologies of these disorders was almost a total void before the turn of the century, and treatment was even more poorly understood. Brain sections revealed little except for the rare findings of Pick's or Alzheimer's diseases,[2] and Ehrlich did not discover the use of arsenicals in the treatment of lues until after 1900.

Since there were so many patients with so little available in terms of etiological diagnosis or specific treatment, the social structure had to develop a method for coping with this new social problem. The answer, in terms of production methodology of the Industrial Revolution, had to lie in terms of low unit cost and mass production, with interchangeable parts. Since no analogue of the production line could diagnose or cure, the warehouse concept had to be invoked. What could be more economical, considerate of the needs of the seemingly non-afflicted members of society, and efficient, as a series of warehouses administered by the state? Each of these warehouses could be built with roughly similar plans and conveniently located in a rural area so that land and labor was not inordinately dear. Assuredly, it was the intention, and the *real* intention, of the designers of these warehouses that there be ample space and humane treatment of the objects to be warehoused, or as they conceived it, hospitalized. Unfortunately, the weight of numbers and the expense of personnel required for the treatment they envisaged, turned the hospitals into warehouses, essentially indistinguishable from those of industry except for the contents.

BIRTH, RISE, and MAINTENANCE

The social phenomena accompanying the rise of industrialization are not only apparent historically, but clearly present today. Poor housing, crowded living conditions, ignorance, anomie, and emptiness with respect to the external world are still the lot of the poor.[4] Identity diffusion, shifting values, geographic mobility, emotional constriction and cognitive rigidity, familial disruption, and emptiness with respect to the inner world appear as the sorrows of the middle classes, having begun with the Industrial Revolution.[6] Thus, there appears to have been ample psychosocial disturbance created during the nineteenth century that would account, in interaction with biological *anlagen,* for the apparent spurt in prevalence and incidence of psychiatric disorders. The process has accelerated with the pace of our civilization.

The realities of social change, however, even when considered in terms of the lack of etiological information and treatment capability of the nineteenth century, do not suffice to explain the rise of the warehousing process in the state hospitals. In contradistinction to that process, the moral therapy of the early nineteenth century represented treatment, and contained many elements of today's treatment techniques, including verbal and activities therapies.[2,7] *It would appear that ideological issues influenced the change from moral treatment to the state hospital system.* There is another axiom implied here, namely that institutional change follows not only from technical advances, but also from ideological influences.

The ideological basis for this development lay in the dual concepts of Social Darwinism and Social Calvinism. Social Darwinism posited a relatively short-term genetic selection of the "survival of the fittest." Rather than reflecting Darwin's ideas that evolution took place over tens and hundreds of millenia, with species selectivity being emphasized, the Social Darwinist advanced the idea that the unfit, including the mentally unfit, were genetic sports who would benefit society by not reproducing. Such people were considered unfit, and hence would be weeded out by natural selection, but within one species and over a short time span; clearly, this was not Darwin's theoretical position, but a convenient interpretation of the times.[8]

There may have been, however, a more powerful ideological underpinning for Social Darwinism in the form of Social Calvinism. In order to define and describe the latter, the issue of Calvinism must be addressed. John Calvin (1509–64) was one of the major figures of the Northern European Reformation accompanying the political break of Germanic Europe from Roman Europe at the end of the Middle Ages. He was, if not the founder of a great deal of social and religious ideology, certainly a very influential transmitter. Specifically, Calvin espoused salvation through grace, in direct and open contradistinction to salvation through works. There was an Elect, a group of people chosen by God to inherit heaven; although others might strive for salvation through good works, they bore little chance of inheriting a heavenly eternity unless they were preordained to do so. The Elect could be distinguished by virtue of their birth, their wealth, their prosperity, their position in society, their health, and similar matters. Calvin's influence was felt in the British Isles as well as on the continent, and it gave rise to English and American Puritanism.[9] In regard to this latter development, Kai Erikson[10] says:

> The first Puritans to reach Massachusetts never saw the contradictions in their theory (nor would they have worried about it if they had) and continued to feel that their position was derived from the soundest logic. But it is important to understand that the essential strength of that logic lay in the conviction that truth had been forever discovered in its entirety. Puritan logic was not a method for learning the truth; it was a rhetorical means for communicating it to others. The twentieth-century reader who tries to feel his way through the mists of Puritan argument may sooner or later decide that it is nothing more than a versatile display of sophistry, but he then must remind himself that men who already *know* the truth have scant need for the niceties of inductive reasoning. The truth as seen by the Puritans was wholly clear. God had chosen an elite to represent Him on earth and to join Him in Heaven. People who belonged to this elite learned of their appointment through the agency of a deep conversion experience, giving them a special responsibility and a special competence to control the destinies of others. People who had never been touched by this moment of grace could have no idea what conversion meant, and thus were simply not qualified to teach the truth or share in the government of men.

Earlier Erikson states that:

> Even Calvin had estimated that only one out of every five persons in an ordinary population was destined for grace.

It is not too difficult then, to posit that, in the mind of the nineteenth-century Calvinist, mental illness and/or poverty were clear indications of not being a member of the Elect and that since salvation was predetermined, it was evident that little could be done for such people. The similarity between the Social Darwinism approach and Calvinism then becomes clear: One posits genetic preordination, while the other invokes spiritual preordination, thereby forming an elegant and consistent dual statement of predestination, one in the material realm, the other in the ideal realm. The consistency is startling.

In light of these considerations, it would appear that the application of Social Darwinism and Social Calvinism to treatment of the mentally ill would certainly allow for the growth of the state hospital system. It would have been economic and ideological folly to have done otherwise, for not even the advances of the Industrial Revolution could be used against *both* nature and the will of God, especially since there was no organ or tissue pathology, and no infectious process found in the majority of cases. The state hospital system was not only economically sound, it was also scientifically correct and morally right.

Once started on its way, with scientific and moral justification, the system built up its own inertial momentum.

The social conditions that provided fertile grounds for breeding mental illness continued and continue today. The ideologies also continued and have only been challenged recently in the light of new advances in etiological understanding. The economy could support the system until recently. However, the phenomena of anomie and identity diffusion are still present. In addition, new populations at risk have appeared, including the aged, abusers of chemical substances, the birth injured, and those with cerebral dysfunction or damage. In addition, the hard core of chronic schizophrenia and severe character amd borderline disturbances remain. The social forces that fostered the growth of the state hospital system remain and the biological components of mental illness appear to have increased in prevalence. Only the ideologies underlying the state hospital system appear to be in question. Consequently, while there is widespread opinion that state hospitals should be discarded, there are apparently significant numbers of people who still require such an institutional system. Elaboration on this matter will be deferred for a later part of this discussion.

DECLINE and COUNTERGROWTH

The seeds of decline of the state hospital system were planted well before its birth. Paradoxically, some growth from these very seeds are currently contributing to the resistance of the system to total disintegration. The social system of Western Europe, as described by thinkers such as Locke in England and Rousseau in France, postulated an essential equality and potential inner true morality in mankind. Locke's *tabula rasa,* the blank state of the individual's mind, and Rousseau's noble savage, the intrinsically good person in a state of nature, could only be contaminated or corrupted by external influences.

Thus, Locke's[11] axiomatic statement, in his "Essay Concerning Human Understanding," goes as follows:

> *All ideas come from sensation or reflection.* -Let us then suppose the mind to be, as we say, white paper, void of all characters, without any ideas; how comes it to be furnished? Whence comes it by that vast store, which the busy and boundless fancy of man has painted on it with an almost endless variety? Whence has it all the materials of reason and knowledge? To this I answer, in one word, from experience. In that all our knowledge is founded, and from that it ultimately derives itself. Our observation, employed either about external sensible objects, or about the internal operations of our minds, perceived and reflected on by ourselves, is that which supplies our understandings with all the materials of thinking. These two are the foundations of knowledge, from whence all the ideas we have, or can naturally have, do spring.

Rousseau[12] concentrated much more on the nature of society and stated axiomatically in the "First Discourse" at Dijon in 1750:

> We cannot reflect on the morality of mankind without contemplating with pleasure the picture of the simplicity which prevailed in the earliest times. This image may be justly compared to a beautiful coast, adorned only by the hands of nature; towards which our eyes are constantly turned, and which we see

receding with regret. While men were innocent and virtuous of their actions, they dwelt together in the same huts; but when they became vicious, they grew tired of such inconvenient onlookers, and banished them to magnificent temples. Finally, they expelled their deities even from these temples, in order to dwell there themselves; or at least the temples of the gods were no longer more magnificent than the palaces of the citizens. This was the height of degeneracy; nor could vice ever be carried to greater lengths than when it was seen, supported, as it were, at the doors of the great, on columns of marble, and graven on Corinthian capitals.

He adds a footnote earlier,

Sovereigns always see with pleasure a taste for the arts of amusement and superfluity, which do not result in the exportation of bullion, increase among their subjects. They very well know that, besides nourishing that littleness of mind which is proper to slavery, the increase of artificial wants only binds so many more chains upon the people. Alexander, wishing to keep the Ichthyophagi in a state of dependence, compelled them to give up fishing, and subsist on the customary food of civilized nations. The American savages, who go naked, and live entirely on the products of the chase, have been always impossible to subdue. What yoke, indeed, can be imposed on men who stand in need of nothing.

Rousseau has been held to be the principle theorist behind the egalitarianism of the French Revolution and its aftermath. Interestingly, the Durants[13] described his early break with the Calvinists of Geneva during the 1760s.

The doctrine of equality, although temporarily suppressed during the same Industrial Revolution it helped to spawn, has once again sprung forth with renewed vigor. As a consequence of the belief in the intrinsic equality of all people, there is a widespread idea that people are all entitled to the same things within their society, or possibly all societies. It follows, therefore, that if the Industrial Revolution has produced goods and afforded services for some, it should do so for all. This has become a principle economic, if not social, tenet of postindustrial society. The crucial issue for psychiatry is, evidently, that the state hospital system was, and is, not seen as equal in quality of service to the private psychiatric hospitals' treatment or to treatment rendered in general hospitals.

The reply to the protest that unequal treatment of different groups of mentally ill persons existed in the United States was the Community Mental Health Centers Act of 1963. This act was presumably based on the most accurate scientific appraisal of the causes and treatment of mental illness then available. The avowedly best scientific theory of its day underlay the reasoning involved in the creation of mental health centers, and can be summarized as follows (as of 1960):

No biological correlates or etiologies for mental illness could be found during the flourishing years of tissue pathology and infectious disease investigations. Moreover, although it appeared that there might be some biochemical components to serious emotional disorder, such components seemed yet unproven or trivial. On the other hand, the various psychodynamic theories of etiology and treatment for almost all psychiatric illnesses were at least relatively consistent internally, if not with each other. Furthermore, they had enormous vogue among many if not most members of several scientific communities. Everyone's mother could be described; it was far more difficult to measure brain function.

The recognition that psychodynamic theories failed to deal with serious psychiatric illness was explained in one of two ways. The first, and more conservative, explanation posited that most identified patients would indeed improve or recover if they all could be treated properly by competent therapists for a sufficiently long time in the proper setting. The alternate explanation lay in positing the inadequacy of the psychodynamic theories and asserted that social processes, particularly those resulting from class orientation, social disruption, and anomie were the real culprits behind the appearance of mental illness.[14] If people were not so poor, if they lived in intact families, if they determined their treatment and who treated them, and if their treatment settings were more humane, then they probably would not become ill and certainly would get better a lot faster if they did become ill. Psychodynamics *might* be of some importance here; biological phenomena were simply dismissed as the ruses of the neo-Calvinists disguised as biochemists.

The question arises: What happened to Social Darwinism and Social Calvinism? The answer, as implied earlier in this discussion, lies in the ideology of our times, when the notion of free will, with its various present-day modification, has once more appeared. In this regard, the following axiom of definition is asserted:

Illness or disorder, whether termed "mental," "psychiatric," or "emotional," as interpreted by the classical social and psychodynamic theories, is seen as a disease of the will. In psychodynamic terms, the identified patient has either *willed* his difficulties on himself, or he has submitted to conflict-engendered anxiety because of some other weakness. In either case, once the conflict is brought to consciousness, and thereby resolved, the identified patient can exercise his free will and become a mature independent adult and a contributor to society. If a sociodynamic frame of reference is invoked, the process is only slightly different; the expression of free will has been suppressed, not by mother, or the superego, but by a repressive society that has not dealt with everyone's intrinsic equality. Once this external pathological suppressor of free will is changed, everyone will then be able to exercise his freedom of choice, with resultant mental health.

Thus, a highly attractive egalitarian ideology, enacted into law, brought about new construction, new jobs, new identities, new hope, and new involvement of the mental health profession in social reform. Intrinsic differences between existential sorrow and depression secondary to object loss, or between biogenic amine abnormality and the grief experienced on losing a child were ignored. It was this systematic neglect of fine differentiation and excess optimism about the benefit of social intervention that led to the inadequate treatment of those persons whose illnesses were chronic and had a significant biological component in their etiologies, despite the widespread use of psychotropic agents.

The dilemma of increasing morbidity in the face of greatly improved treatment capability, both social and biological, has become readily apparent. The collective psychodynamics contributing toward this condition can be described as follows:

All psychiatric illness is caused either by biological factors or by sociofamilial factors. If biological factors are considered predominant, then this is tantamount to saying that there exists a significant number of human beings who have been foreordained by God or nature to suffer from such predominantly biological disease. In the Calvinist tradition, such people demonstrate the clear will of God that they are not members of the Elect. It would be inappropriate to attempt treatment, because it would be unsuccessful. This is expressed in pseudoquestions of house staff such as "Is it worth treating this patient?" or in the mandate of cost-control boards who suggest the "ordering of priorities," or by the euphemism "triage." Utilizing the rationalizations of "economy," "suitability for treatment," or similar phrases, those whom society would deem as preordained to illness are regarded, consciously or unconsciously, as not worthy of treatment. Therefore, the general concept has evolved that biological etiology should not be invoked, since it implies inferiority and untreatability. A conflict model of illness becomes preferable, even if inappropriately applied to some people, because in it lies hope. As people are treated in accordance with this conflict model, however, therapeutic failures appear; the sicker population increases, and the state hospital system once more becomes necessary, either as a thing in itself, or as such an economically viable substitute as "skilled nursing facilities" that "accept" people labeled as "mildly to moderately psychiatrically ill." There has been a repression or suppression of the concept of biological disease because in the

Calvinist scheme, this concept has been equated to exclusion from the Elect and hence to untreatability.

The net result has been that the mental health professions have espoused salvation through works, such as represented by the psychotherapies, pharmacotherapy, and short-term hospitalization, while ignoring the hard fact that there are many people who are very ill as a consequence of the interaction of biological propensity and social processes. The state hospital system has undergone dismantling and piecemeal reconstruction as a consequence, and the difficulties remain.

CONCLUSION

It would appear that there exists a considerable number of identified patients who have been so traumatized by life experiences, or more frequently, who suffer from such severe biological disorder and social anomie that they require intermediate or long-term humane care in a semisheltered or sheltered setting. It is clear from examination of any set of patients who are seriously ill, that there are significant numbers of sick persons living in our society. If it is recognized that even those who are seriously ill are nevertheless equal in their right to care, and that such care may not be wholly "economical," then there may be a viable, humane state hospital system, or if not, a place within the community for the severely and chronically disabled.

REFERENCES

1. Galbraith, J. K.: *The Affluent Society.* Boston: Houghton Mifflin, 1958.

2. Zilboorg, G.: *A History of Medical Psychology.* New York: George Braziller, 1975.

3. Goffman, E.: *Asylums: Essays on the Social Situation of Mental Patients and Other Inmates.* Chicago: Aldine Publishing Co., 1961.

4. Wilensky, H. L. & Lebeauz, C. N.: *Industrial Society: Social Welfare.* New York: The Free Press, 1965.

5. Greenberg, I. M.: *General Systems: Social and Biological Interactions.* (Submitted for publication).

6. Ericson, E.: *Childhood and Society.* New York: Norton, 2nd ed., 1950.

7. Ackerknecht, E.: *A Short History of Modern Psychiatry.* (S. Wolff, trans.), Hafner Press, Distributed by Collier-Macmillan, Riverside, New Jersey, 1969.

8. McNeill, W.: *Rise of the West: A History of the Human Community.* (Collector's Edition Series). Chicago: University of Chicago Press, 1968.

9. Smith, L. B.: "John Calvin" in *Makers of Modern Thought.* New York: American Heritage, 1972.

10. Erikson, K. T.: *Wayward Puritans: A Study in The Sociology of Deviance.* New York: Wiley, 1966.

11. Locke, J.: "An Essay Concerning Human Understanding" in *The English Philosophers from Bacon to Mill.* New York: Modern Library, 1939.

12. Rousseau, J. J.: *A Discourse on the Arts and Sciences in the Social Contract and Discourses.* (G. D. H. Cole, trans.), New York: Dutton, 1950.

13. Durant, W. & Durant, A.: *Rousseau and Revolution: The Story of Civilization.* New York: Simon and Schuster, 1967.

14. Scheff, T. J., ed.: *Mental Illness and Social Processes.* New York: Harper and Row, 1967.

Chapter 3

MISSION IMPOSSIBLE: EFFECTS OF BUREAUCRATIC RIGIDITY

A. Anthony Arce, M.D.

The mission, organization, administration, and fate of public programs are largely the result of a "continuing process of bargaining, pressuring, inducing, bribing, supervision, demonstrating, harassing, encouraging, and publicizing"[1] that takes place among governments, service agencies, professionals, and more recently, the public at large. Social problems may be identifiable and quantifiable. The required professionals, approaches or interventions to deal with social problems may be ascertainable. The professional may entertain a variety of fantasies as to the impact of his or her expertise on the formulation of policy or the shaping of delivery systems. While the professional's influence may not be inconsequential, what is ultimately feasible programmatically is the result of political and bureaucratic decisions.

The purpose of this chapter is to explore in rather bold fashion the implications of bureaucratic rigidities on mental health program implementation in the context of the new mission for the state hospital within the mental health services delivery system. My perspective is that of a former state hospital director who is now a community mental health center director.

A New Role for State Hospitals

Toward the end of the nineteenth century, responsibility for the care of the mentally ill was assumed by state governments and until the 1960s the mental health delivery system was dominated by the state mental hospital. Overpopulated and understaffed, socially and geographically isolated from the communities from which their patients came, and subject to the constraints of increasingly complex governmental bureaucracies, these state hospitals, nevertheless, fulfilled faithfully and, perhaps even well, their assigned mission of providing custodial care for those whom society could not accept.

In the 1950s, a reorientation in the approach to the care of the mentally ill occurred in the direction of community care as opposed to institutional care. The introduction of the neuroleptic agents for the first time gave rise to the hope that the chronically ill, state hospital patient could be treated in the community. The resident population of public mental hospitals peaked at over one-half million in 1965 and then began a steady decline, which continues today though at a much reduced rate. From the perspective of the state hospital system, this decline in population could only lead to an improvement in the ratio between staff and patients, which in turn would result in the ability of these same staffs to deliver quality therapeutic care instead of merely custodial care.

The development of community mental health and the passage of the Community Mental Health Centers Act in 1963 were interpreted as administering the *coup de grace* to the state hospital system. One began to read with increasing frequency about the phasing out of the state hospitals.[2,3] However, within a decade it became amply clear that the dire predictions of doom had been premature.[4] The California experience began to raise serious doubts as to the feasibility and desirability of the ultimate closing of all state hospitals. By 1973, California had reduced its state hospital population by 80 per cent and the proposed closing of the hospitals seemed an achievable goal. A committee of the California senate was charged with the responsibility for investigating the merits of the proposal. During extensive hearings, the committee heard evidence that community mental health programs were not effective in caring for the chronically ill discharged from state hospitals. It concluded that "state hospitals continue to serve as an indispensable component of the mental health system. . . ."[5] Essentially, the issue that had to be faced was whether the "involuntary communitization"[6] of state hospital patients leads to any significant degree of improvement in the quality of their lives.[7]

Statistical analyses of patient movements have revealed that in the face of decreasing census in state hospitals, admissions to these facilities have actually increased, with readmissions rising proportionately more than first admissions. Obviously, community mental health centers are screening out former state hospital patients as "untreatable" and these patients continue to be the responsibility of the state hospital system. While community mental health services represent undeniable progress in the delivery of services to those in need, they are not the panacea promised by the proponents and advocates of the community mental health movement. In fact, it appears that state hospital care will continue to be an essential component of the total delivery system for the foreseeable future.

The anticipated demise of the state hospital as a result of developments in the community mental health movement and the passage of the Community Mental Health Centers Act thus has not come to pass. Instead, increasingly, state mental hospitals have come to be viewed as integral parts of comprehensive community mental health services in full and equal partnership with community agencies. To accomplish this new mission, state hospitals are expected to undertake the implementation of innovative relationships with other community agencies in an effort to avoid duplication of services, insure continuity of care, and increase the more effective utilization of shrinking resources.

In New York State, the Department of Mental Hygiene sponsored legislation aimed at fostering this process of collaboration. The aim of the Unified Services Bill was to create a single system of services by binding the disparate elements of several service systems—state, local, and private—with sufficient strength to create new program identities for all the involved agencies and their personnel. For instance, it might be preferable for the local community mental health board and the state hospital to develop a single jointly administered and staffed program than to merely coordinate the activities of their separate programs through mutual referrals, the sharing of information or other less binding devices. Such notions raised numerous questions concerning accountability, the relationship between the state and local bureaucracies, the problems generated by the sharing of staff belonging to two separate civil service systems, and the abdication of a measure of state government authority over its facilities in the service of more rational relationships at the local level. Although only 5 counties out of 62 elected to utilize the unified services funding plan in which the state would pay 87 per cent of all local costs and the counties would pay only 13 per cent, the joint planning aspects of the legislation were undertaken almost without exception but with only minimal degrees of success. Efforts to plan and implement such collaborative programs between the state hospital and its community have been impeded by bureaucratic obstacles.

BUREAUCRACY AND THE MENTAL HEALTH FIELD

Bureaucracies are relatively modern social inventions developed as a reaction against the managerial chaos of the early days of the Industrial Revolution. Managerial practices in those days were characterized by personal subjugation, despotism, cruelty and capricious judgment. The bureaucractic structure was intended to provide a sense of order and rationality in the organization and the management of the industrial firm.

At the turn of the century, Max Weber,[8] a German sociologist, described the fundamental characteristics of the bureaucratic structure. They are (1) a division of labor based on functional specialization; (2) a well defined hierarchy of authority; (3) a system of rules covering the rights and duties of employees; (4) a system of procedures for dealing with work situations; (5) impersonality of interpersonal relationships; and (6) promotion and selection based on technical competence.

However, in contrast, most people perceive bureaucracies as incredibly encrusted machines that are bound by traditional ways of doing things, are populated with superiors and subordinates who lack competence, and are managed by means of arbitrary and zany rules. According to Bennis,[9] the many criticisms of bureaucracy "outnumber and outdo the ninety-five theses tacked on the church door at Wittenberg." Some examples: bureaucracies develop conformity and group-think. They modify personality structure so that people become and reflect the dull, gray, conditioned organization man. Bureaucracies do not take into account the informal organization and cannot cope with emergency or unanticipated problems. Their systems of control and authority are hopelessly outdated. Bureaucracies cannot assimilate the influx of new technology, and they thwart communication and innovative ideas by means of hierarchical divisions.

The chief characteristic of bureaucracies is the preoccupation with rules. Official compilations of rules and regulations, policies and procedures manuals, job descriptions and staffing pattern prescriptions pursue the unsuspecting administrator at every turn; all are designed to tell him why something cannot be done. In any organization, individual units have different functions, face different needs, and operate in different environments. They tend to acquire different characteristics, norms, and values. Rules that may appear rational from a general perspective may pose obstacles to individual units in the fulfillment of their mission. Furthermore, procedures for dealing with work situations may not be applicable across units which vary significantly in goals, functions, and missions. What is functional for one may be dysfunctional for another. In their preoccupation with ensuring standards of performance and functioning, of protecting against abuses and irregularities, and of maintaining order and equality, bureaucracies lose sight of the need for flexibility and adaptability to changing situations and needs.

Flexibility and adaptability are especially relevant when the interorganizational field, that is, the environment in which an organization operates, is in a state of flux as a result of modifications in technology, changing sociopolitical patterns, scarcity of resources, and so on. Such interorganizational fields have been called "disturbed reactive" or "turbulent"[10] and are characterized by change, not only in the relationships among members of the field but also in the nature and defining characteristics of the field.

Such is the state of the community mental health services field at the present time. Among its salient features are: increased scope of services; larger and more diverse staffs; complex organizational patterns featuring multi-unit systems coordinated with other services; sophisticated management information and evaluation; shifting patterns of government involvement and responsibility among federal, state, and local levels; greater community involvement and increased sensitivity to change.[11] The capacity of state mental health programs to change in response to the articulated needs of the society around them may be the single most important determinant of their growth and viability. And it is precisely in their capacity for flexibility/adaptability that bureaucracies are most wanting.

BUREAUCRATIC OBSTACLES TO PROGRAM INNOVATION

Government bureaucracies especially are ponderous machines locked in statutory and regulatory devices for the purpose of the managing of public funds. They consist of a system of interlocking bureaucracies each with its own territorial assignment and zealously guarded prerogatives. Such service bureaucracies as the departments of mental hygiene, health, and social services are subject to the contraints imposed by such regulatory bureaucracies as the civil service commission for personnel management, the office of general services for the procurement of space for community programs, and the department of audit and control for evaluating program efficiency. In other words, upon the already cumbersome bureaucractic apparatuses of the service organizations are superimposed those of the regulatory agencies. The result is a system so encumbered with checks and balances that it responds slowly to changing needs and makes progress difficult. The system is unable to absorb creativity and innovation because of its heavy reliance on formal structures and its dependence on hierarchies of authority and on procedures for reporting and accountability

In most states, the state mental hospital system continues to be the repository of the bulk of the public funds expended for mental health services. In New York State, for instance, the direct state contribution to community programs still averages less than 10 per cent of the state's expenditures for mental health. Expenditures for the operation of state facilities for the mentally ill and the developmentally disabled amount to 83 per cent of the total operating budget of the Department of Mental Hygiene. Between 1965 and 1972, hospital populations decreased by 40 per cent but expenditures for hospital operations rose by 81 per cent. The increased emphasis on a community approach to the care of the mentally ill has resulted in a decided shift in the locus of care from hospital to community but not in a concurrent shift in resources.

As the state hospital moves into its new partnership with the community it serves, it brings to its relationships with other agencies a decided advantage: its still considerable resources. In spite of their growing resentment at the inequities in funding vis-à-vis the levels of service expected of them in what they perceive as a one-way street, community agencies are often eager to enter into collaborative agreements of one sort or another with the state hospital, especially in view of decreasing federal involvement in financing community mental health services. It is not, therefore, unreasonable for them to expect that the state hospital resources will be equally as available for "communitization" as the patients have been. Such expectations, however, are not infrequently dashed against a stone wall at one or another level of the state bureaucracy because of "the need for accountability in the expenditure of public funds," "the possibility of exposing the state to negligence or liability claims," or the inability to find a rule that covers the specific arrangement proposed.

The hospital, of course, has the option of developing a state operated program in the community. Besides the fact that this is not in keeping with the partnership concept and is presumably frowned upon by the policy makers, the establishment of a state-operated program requires the procurement of space in the community through a process so lengthy and cumbersome as to frustrate even the most patient and hardy among administrators. The Office of General Services, which in New York State is the bureaucracy empowered to secure and lease space for state operations, has recently streamlined its procedures for the finding and leasing of space from 42 to 40 steps. This, however, has not appreciably shortened the lead time required from the submission of the request to final occupancy from the usual 10–12 months. In the meantime, conditions may change on any number of fronts requiring a revision of the proposed program which will only further delay implementation.

But it is in the area of personnel management that state bureaucratic systems have demonstrated their weakness in the recruitment, development, distribution, and maintenance of the skilled manpower needed to serve the people entrusted to the care of state mental health systems.

The achievement of organizational goals depends essentially on the strengths and weaknesses of the people who populate the organization. The quality of mental health care is a reflection of the staff who conduct the treatment program, their numbers, their experience, and their human qualities.

In the past, it was possible to operate large custodial institutions with quantitatively and qualitatively substandard staffs of professionals and nonprofessionals. The quality of care and the prevailing conditions at such institutions may have been terrible but those facilities were socially and geographically isolated from their communities and, therefore, tolerated. Staff organization in such institutions was characterized by, among other things, caste-like divisions of line staff into hierarchically ranked categories with clearly delineated roles and responsibilities at each level; a lack of mobility among staff categories; and the phenomenon of multiple subordination, in which each successive lower level of staff was expected to respond to requests and orders from all levels above. Newcomers to the staff ultimately became institutionalized like their patients and settled into comfortable routines within the established order. Under these circumstances, civil service practices were seldom, if ever, challenged.

But in recent years, the emphasis has been on staffs characterized by organization into teams more ecumenical in both composition and function. This has been associated with less concern for hierarchies, an increase in role-blurring among professional disciplines, and a rapid expansion in the utilization, in a variety of roles, of community mental health workers, otherwise and more condescendingly referred to as paraprofessionals. Traditional civil service job descriptions and classifications have not been modified sufficiently as yet to take into account these changing patterns in program needs and staff utilization. As a result, state hospital directors must frequently disregard civil service rules, regulations, and procedures in an effort to meet their program requirements.

Furthermore, in the community, each worker, regardless of discipline and rank, operates with a high degree of autonomy and privacy, constantly dealing with new problems, contingencies, and situations that have not been anticipated and for which there are no established or prescribed procedures. The worker must rely on his or her judgment, ingenuity, and experience in dealing with such unforeseen circumstances. This generates not only enthusiasm and commitment to the job, but also a significant degree of pride in the performance of work that in turn enhances self-esteem. Exposure of state hospital custodial staffs to these kinds of rewards has resulted in a significant increase in pressure for opportunities for advancement as well as "salary blurring." Efforts at implementing patient care career ladders have been hampered by adherence to traditional pyramidal staffing arrangements. As for salary blurring, in traditional bureaucratic fashion, everyone plays ostrich; if one doesn't look at it, it will go away.

The ultimate regulatory bureaucracy in the entire state system is the department of audit and control whose task it is to conduct audits of the operations of the service bureaucracies. Audit and control, of course, is itself immune from such scrutiny. The purpose of these management analyses is to ascertain whether policies and procedures are being properly applied, to determine operating efficiency and level of employee productivity, and to assure the effective usage of available resources. I quote from a personal but official communication: "The overriding objective is to provide a factually correct, balanced, and constructive report which will be of assistance to management in increasing efficiency, economy and effectiveness of operations."

The department of audit and control is staffed with individuals whose primary training and concern is fiscal, i.e., accounting clerks and accountants; and while their function is essentially to ensure that public funds have not been misappropriated or misused, in recent years they have increasingly subsumed program evaluation functions. We are thus faced with the absurdity of having nonclinicians making clinical judgments on quality of care. This is no mean feat since, even for clinicians, evaluation of mental health care in general is beset with numerous pitfalls given the state of our knowledge, the incredible intricacy of the problems, the difficulties in defining what we mean by "success" in terms of outcome and the need to control numerous variables. But the ultimate regulatory bureaucracy is ready to tell us precisely how to do it.

New and different kinds of interorganizational relationships are needed to accomplish the goal of successfully treating the mentally ill in the community through single systems of services. Inasmuch as the task of managing these new multiunit systems has been equated with conducting a symphony orchestra, it is conceivable that a report from a department of audit and control would read something like this:

MANAGEMENT ANALYSIS OF CANARSIE
SYMPHONY

For considerable periods of time the four oboe players have nothing to do. Their numbers should be reduced, and the work spread more evenly over the whole of the concert, thus eliminating peaks of activity. All of the 12 first violins were playing identical notes; this seems unnecessary duplication. The staff of this section should be drastically cut. If a large volume of sound is required it could be obtained by means of electronic amplification apparatus. Much effort was absorbed in the playing of semiquavers. This seems to be an excessive refinement. It is recommended that all notes should be rounded up to the nearest quaver. If this were done, it would be possible to use trainees and lower-grade operatives more extensively. There seems to be too much repetition of some musical passages. Scores should be drastically pruned. No useful purpose is served by repeating on the horns a passage that has already been played by the strings. It is estimated that if all redundant passages were eliminated, the whole concert time of the two hours could be reduced to twenty minutes and there would be no need for an intermission.[12]

Conclusion

To summarize, the redefinition of this mission of the state hospital as a partner in the delivery of mental health services poses an exciting challenge for both administrators and staff. The achievement of this goal will undoubtedly revitalize the state hospital system. However, the full actualization of this new role is being hindered, if not prevented, by the oppressive rigidity of the multilayered bureaucracy that is the state governmental system. Unless these obstacles are modified so as to permit greater flexibility in operationalizing the new mandate for these facilities, the state hospital system is doomed to remain a second-class, backup system.

References

1. Connery, R. H., et al.: *The Politics of Mental Health.* New York: Columbia University Press, 1968.

2. Stewart A., Lafave, H. G., Grunberg F., et al.: "Problems in phasing out a large public psychiatric hospital." *American Journal of Psychiatry* 125: 82–88, 1968.

3. Hecker, A. C.: "The demise of large state hospitals." *Hospital Community Psychiatry* 21: 261–263, 1970.

4. Lamb, H. R., Goertzel, V.: "The demise of the state hospitals: A premature obituary?" *Archives of General Psychiatry* 26:489–495, June 1972.

5. Final report to the California legislature of the Senate Select Committee on Proposed Phaseout of State Hospital Services. Sacramento, California, March 15, 1974.

6. Rachlin, S.: "With liberty and psychosis for all." *Psychiatric Quarterly* 48: 410–420, 1974.

7. Reich, R.: "Care of the chronically mentally ill—a national disgrace." *American Journal of Psychiatry* 130:911–912, 1973.

8. Weber, M.: *The Theory of Social and Economic Organization.* New York, Oxford University Press, 1947.

9. Bennis, W. G.: "Beyond Bureaucracy," *Trans-Action* 2(5):31–35, 1965.

10. Emery, S. E., & Trist, E. L.: "The causal texture of organizational environment." *Human Relations* 18:21–32, 1965.

11. Feldman, S.: *The Administration of Mental Health Services.* Springfield, Ill.: Charles C. Thomas, 1973.

12. Greenblatt M., Cited in Proceedings, 1976 midwinter meeting, American Association of Directors of Psychiatry Residency Training, New Orleans, La., January 16–18, 1976, p.3.

Chapter 4

THE PUBLIC HOSPITAL SYSTEM AS A NEXUS BETWEEN GOVERNMENT AND THE UNIVERSITY

Israel Zwerling, M.D., Ph.D.

The detonation of an atomic bomb over Hiroshima on August 6, 1945, destroyed forever any lingering illusions about the separability of society and science. Concern about the mutual responsibilities of each to the other—i.e., the social obligations of the scientist and in turn the obligations of government to the scientific community—did not of course begin with that mushroom cloud, but what had tended to be a remote and passionless issue became at once a matter of survival urgency. The initial absorption, understandably enough, was specifically with the physicist. Over the years, and most acutely in the last decade, more and more of the academic community has crowded onto center stage in these discussions as the geneticist, immunologist, demographer, petrochemist, economist, behavior therapist, and psychosurgeon, among others, have been perceived as possessing an expertise of critical or even survival implications to society. It is quite clear at this point that the issue applies equally to the biological, behavioral, medical, and social scientist, as to the physicist, and that the problem addressed can most appropriately be broadly stated as the nature of the relationship between government and the university.

It seems equally clear that a very appropriate locus at which to examine this interface is the public mental health system, including the state mental hospital. Relationships range across a broad spectrum. At one extreme are those situations in which scattered universities, unrelated to each other or to a particular mental health center or hospital, have trained the various specialists who happen to work in that center or hospital. At the other extreme is the community mental health center or the state mental hospital that is operated by a university and itself serves as an educational center. Many aspects of the interface are patently more visible in the latter instance, but they are no less real in the former, and indeed some of the failures of the university to meet what I suggest are its obligations to society are most starkly evident in the isolated and unaffiliated state hospital.

The period since World War II has witnessed a massive shift in the expectation of what, broadly, may be described as society's responsibility to man. The principle that health and health care are human rights, and not privileges available for purchase, has been one feature of the profound social change, along and intertwined with the principles embodied in such endeavors as the civil rights movement, the War Against Poverty, and the Peace Corps. Societal responsibility for health care rapidly brought with it the demand that the university participate, and this is nowhere more directly presented than in the Report of the Carnegie Commission on Higher Education:[1]

> The Commission recommends that university health service centers should be responsible, in their respective geographic areas, for coordinating the education of health care personnel and for cooperation with other community agencies in improving the organization of health care delivery. Their educational and research programs should become more concerned with problems of health care delivery and the social and economic environment of health care.

Now the systems of state mental hospitals long antedate current pressures for a national health insurance program, and universities were responsive to public opinion and to the needs of the job marketplace long before the report of the Carnegie Commission. There has been ample time for the development of a relatively stable relationship between government and the university. In a contextual setting in which rapid advances in knowledge about community and hospital care of the mentally ill are occurring, and pressures both for public and for university responsibility for the ill are increasing, the public mental health system has become a uniquely suitable laboratory for examining the relationship between government and the university. The most cursory inspection reveals that the relationship is in many ways seriously flawed, riddled with failures on the part of each to meet the needs of the other. I would like to describe briefly some of the failures, discuss some of their possible causes, and offer some suggestions about how the relationship might be improved.

The most serious flaw, in my view, is the failure of academia to prepare professional mental health workers for careers in the public mental health sector and to promote research relevant to that sector. Time does not permit the full delineation of this issue, which has been detailed in a recent publication in which I participated[2] and which I commend to your attention. The shift from custodial care for the mentally ill in geographically remote fortresses to active treatment in community-based centers and hospitals in the past two decades is but one manifestation of a revolution in both concept and practice brought about by the community mental health movement. We are confronted by unaccustomed numbers of patients, from unaccustomed socioeconomic and ethnic population groups, with unaccustomed disorders, and in unaccustomed age groupings. Communities challenge the neocolonial pattern of bringing services to them without consulting them, and they challenge much of our diagnostic system as a labeling device for blaming the victims of an oppressive social structure. Mental health

professionals are engaged in unaccustomed patterns of work—
as team members, rather than as solo practitioners, and with
unaccustomed allies—with sociologists and demographers and
political scientists. The conceptual exclusivity enjoyed by psychodynamic theory has been broadened not only to the neurobi-
ological systems level but to the family, the community, the
social class, and the culture as determinants of behavior. Programs for prevention and community consultation have begun
to receive public fiscal support—inadequate, to be sure, but
representing a significant fraction of the total allocation for
mental health. The response of the universities to all this change
has been a thunderous silence, or more accurately, perhaps, a
barely audible squeak. The Report of the Task Force on Delivery of Psychiatric Services to Poverty Areas,[3] for example,
notes that "By the time the (psychiatry) resident gets into the
community, his training has emphasized intensive service to
limited numbers of predominantly middle-class patients utilizing a dynamic diadic approach." This very succinct report lists
20 major "Recommendations for Study." Graduate programs
in clinical psychology and in psychiatric social work have been
similarly unresponsive. Government—in the form of creden-
tialing procedures and the associated licensure and Board ex-
aminations—has in its turn provided no pressure on the
university to accommodate to a societal need now at least 20
years old.

If the major default of the university to government has
been the failure to focus meaningful educational and research
attention to an urgent social need—a fault of *omission*—then
not too far behind is the rip-off of resources intended for public
service for nonsocietal university intersts, a fault of *commission*.
Here I am treading on sensitive ground, and the data I can offer
are anecdotal and personal, rather than objective and statistical.
What immediately comes to mind is an episode early in my
accepting the directorship of the Bronx State Hospital in October 1966. There were then 14 fully populated wards of geriatric
"patients," a very small fraction of whom had been admitted

for a treatable psychiatric illness. Standards for the admission of patients were then carefully spelled out, and in a very short time I received a letter from the chairman of the department of medicine of the Albert Einstein College of Medicine asking me to please unblock his department's accustomed channel for the disposition of elderly patients admitted to the university's teaching hospital with stroke or heart disease who no longer could serve any of his teaching needs. I wrote back enclosing a copy of my guidelines for admission, and added the admonition that I intended to call to the attention of the ethics committee of our county medical society the next instance of a patient sent over from the college teaching hospital who died within 24 hours after arrival. When I left the Bronx State Hospital seven years later there were three geriatric wards, and I understand there are now, four years later, only two.

I do not propose that this is representative of the most flagrant exploitation of government by university—the many instances of the deployment of funds, space, laboratories, and other resources of a public mental health system for university purposes totally unrelated to the mental health needs of the community, about which I know, I do not feel free to discuss. I cannot refrain from adding one additional personal experience. Shortly after assuming my present position as chairman of the Department of Mental Health Sciences of the Hahnemann Medical College and Hospital, I was approached by Dr. Daniel Blain with a request that I help him locate a suitable director of training for the Philadelphia State Hospital. He reviewed for me the sad history of the exploitation of that hospital by several of the Philadelphia medical schools in past efforts at establishing liaison relationships, and appealed to my recent experience as director of a state hospital to change this pattern. I asked my staff for recommendations of possible candidates for the position of director of training at Philadelphia State Hospital, pointing out that I was new to the area and did not yet know the professional community. One of the senior staff members submitted a recommendation. Entirely coincidentally the psychiatrist he had proposed called that day to ask if there were any teaching positions available in my department. I set up an appointment to meet with him and triumphantly called my colleague to report the bit of serendipity, only to be told "Oh, God! We don't want *him* in *our* department!" At the following meeting of the executive staff of my department, I reported this incident and stated simply, "Don't any of you ever do this to me again." We did, parenthetically, provide a superb director of training to the Philadelphia State Hospital from our faculty.

Government, in its turn, has been no less unmindful of the character and needs of the university The incompatibility of traditional bureaucratic process of government with university process has been a major source of friction at their interface, and a very recent personal experience illustrates this point quite well. For reasons not germane to the present point—though representative of an issue to which I will shortly return—the legislature in Pennsylvania voted a precipitous cut in the budget of the Eastern Pennsylvania Psychiatric Institute (EPPI), a state hospital created to provide a resource for training and research in mental health. I was asked to chair a committee that was to recommend to the State Commissioner of Mental Health how the budget cut was to be implemented, based on the merits of the various investigative and educational programs. A group of specialists, expert in the particular fields of study represented by the service and research divisions and departments at EPPI, was recruited, and the programs at EPPI were intensively reviewed, including a careful scrutiny of the publications of each unit and interviews with each unit chief. On the basis of this survey, a careful priority list was established and submitted to the commissioner. We were profusely thanked for what, in all modesty, was indeed an excellent review—and the state proceeded to ignore the recommendations and, in response to union pressure, to eliminate positions primarily on the basis of seniority. Productive scientists, engaged in fruitful research in the front lines of the concerns of the public mental health system were terminated; unit chiefs employed as full-time researchers who had not published a single contribution in a decade were retained. Instances in which, similarly, the state employee's unions or the civil service apparatus presented insurmountable obstacles to the missions agreed upon by government and the university can be cited literally by the score. Teaching and research programs, by their very nature, demand a degree of flexibility beyond what government as a rule can provide.

A particular aspect of this general issue that tends to be especially troublesome to government-university relationships in the public mental health system is the inability of government to provide the assurance of continued support for the duration of a program, which is so frequently required. The decision of the legislature to slash the EPPI budget is a case in point; many of the programs, as has been indicated, did not merit support, but this was of course not known by the legislators and in any event was not corrected by their action; they voted on the basis of their priorities for the state, and the result was that, with two-weeks' notice, more than 150 scientists, virtually all with faculty appointments in a Philadelphia medical school were simply terminated. The more usual experience is a more gradual withering away of programs—my department at the Hahnemann Medical College in Philadelphia now enjoys having an outstanding psychiatrist as director of our community mental health center because New York State had, through budget cuts, made it impossible for him to maintain the productive affiliation he had developed between the state hospital he directed there and a first-rate university department of psychiatry. Again, scores of instances can be cited in which the government was unable to capitalize on the availability of a university program because it could not guarantee support for the duration of the program.

There are inherent strains in a government-university relationship that are readily apparent; they derive from the differences in the essential nature and purpose of each, and they account for at least some of the difficulties I have noted. The government, ideally, is concerned with what is *right* for the greatest number of its citizens; its decisions are essentially moral and are rarely the product of experimental research. The university, on the contrary, is ideally concerned with what is *true,* rather than what is right; it is morally neutral. The government is *realistic;* it accepts that at any given moment in time there are unsolved problems and unresolved conflicts, and that compromises are necessary if the society is to get on with its work. The university is *optimistic* and operates with the conviction that knowledge is indefinitely perfectible and that more knowledge is necessarily better than less. Holton[4] has reviewed the basic difference in philosophical orientation between the person-oriented government and the nonperson-orientation of the scientist; the latter may be studying people, but the pursuit itself tends to be "objective" and impersonal. The composite value orientations of the scientist and university are then in fundamental ways in opposition to those of government, and this stands in the way of meaningful dialogue. A clear example of this is the report of Delahunt,[5] who has noted some of his experiences as a member of the Massachusetts legislature in attempting to develop legislation designed to curb or restrain biomedical research; essentially he blames the scientists' failure to grasp the legislative process for his own misdirected but successful efforts to obtain passage of a bill prohibiting fetal research.

There are, at the same time, in the arena of the public mental health system, significant political or power issues that unite government and the university. Neither has a record of which they can be proud for concern for the underprivileged and minority groups who constitute a significant segment of recipients of public mental health services. I would hypothesize that collaboration between the two entities in the areas of research concerning diseases of the affluent is significantly better than in mental illness (or in sickle-cell disease); one need only contrast the degree to which the Nixon administration set out to eliminate federal support for mental health training and community mental health services with their maintenance of support for heart disease, stroke, and cancer. The university, on its part, has reflected very similar priorities—contrast, for example, the all-out response of academia to Sputnik with its no-response to the community mental health movement. Ours is not necessarily a society for all the people, notwithstanding our traditional rhetoric. Sieghart,[6] reporting on the deliberations of a cross-disciplinary committee in England whose goal is "to devise practial means, *within the framework of the existing social system,* for the performance of the social obligations of scientists" (emphasis mine), reports that their committee considered "radical—if not revolutionary—reform of the entire social system" and discarded this as a solution because "We do not believe that revolution in Great Britain is likely in the long run to be more effective than reform in improving the quality of life enjoyed by most people." Having, however, rejected revolution as a means, presumably in favor of reform as a means, the end somehow disappears as well, and rather than social reform, the recommendations of the committee for necessary actions fall entirely upon the shoulders of the scientists themselves. Thus, for example, he writes, "where there is an urgent social need for a piece of research, or the development of a technology there may well be a special responsibility, resting on those scientists who are specially qualified to undertake such work, rather than some other work of lower social value, even though such a course of action may bring them a lesser reward in earnings or fame."

The dilemma of the socially (or governmentally) oriented scientists or academician is a very distressing one. Holton[4] indicates that there is respectable anecdotal reason to think that a frequent psychodynamic sequence leading to a career choice in science is the promise of an escape from the uncertainties, injustices, and inequalities of everyday life into a world of defined, lawful, and elegant simplicity and lucidity. This is certainly consistent with the finding of Roe[7] that of the 64 leading scientists she studied, only four played any active role in any political or civic organization. Holton estimates that "The fraction of U.S. scientists active ... (to the point of helping to formulate or administer science policy on matters of explicit societal concerns, or even writing or teaching occasionally on the topic) is of the order of one per cent."

Holton[4] and Sieghart[6] both emphasize the crucial role played by those scientists who transcend the isolating forces and enter actively in community or government affairs, and the contributions that such persons can make are self-evident. However, my own view is that it is unlikely that change in the relationship between the university and government in the arena of public mental health will come in any significant measure from the university. To be sure, some will: the mode of work increasingly demanded of professionals in community mental health must inevitably force some change in the training institutions, through staff simultaneously serving as faculty, through the experience provided to students and trainees assigned to public mental health programs for field placement, and through the market place. These changes predictably will permit community mental health centers and state hospitals to become more selective in recruiting new staff as alternative positions in traditional programs diminish. But this is likely to prove a painfully slow process. It rather seems to me that more rapid and more profound change will follow upon community demands—through government—for the training of new professionals. I do not think that the "age of consumerism" is fading away; I see it instead as having now only begun the process whereby citizens, through government, will demand participation in the making of all policy relevant to the quality of life in their communities. I have the happy fantasy that it will be in response to community pressure that the university will some day recruit and train scientists who will be both person- and nonperson-oriented, and that the humanist-scientist of the university, in interaction with a political scientist as the representative of government, will negotiate a new relationship between government and the university in the area of public mental health. I also have the unhappy fantasy that we may not be very far from a radical and explosive resolution of the current dilemmas in which chunks of the baby may be flushed away with the dirty bath water. The courts in Rouse, and Wyatt, and Donaldson, and scores of other decisions are sending loud messages about the state of affairs in the public mental health system. I hope that government and the university take heed.

REFERENCES

1. Carnegie Commission on Higher Education: *Higher Education and the Nation's Health.* New York: McGraw-Hill, 1970.

2. Alvarez R., et al.: *Racism, Professionalism and Elitism: Barriers to Community Mental Health.* New York: Jason Aronson, 1976.

3. American Psychiatric Association: *Report of the Task Force on Delivery of Psychiatric Services to Poverty Areas* (mimeographed). Washington, D.C.: *APA* author, October 1973.

4. Holton, G.: *Scientific Optimism and Societal Concerns.* Hastings Center Report, Institute of Society, Ethics and the Life Science, Vol. 5, Hastings-on-Hudson, New York: 1975.

5. Delahunt, W. D.: *Biomedical Research: A View from the State Legislature.* Hastings Center Report, Institute of Society, Ethics and the Life Science, Vol. 6, Hastings-on-Hudson, New York: 1976.

6. Sieghart, P.: *The Social Obligations of the Scientist.* Hastings Center Report, Institute of Society Ethics and the Life Science, Vol. 1, Hastings-on-Hudson, New York: 1973.

7. Roe A.: *The Making of a Scientist.* New York: Dodd, Mead, 1952.

Chapter 5

THE FILTRATION BED PHENOMENON AND ITS RELATION TO STAFF COMPETENCE AND QUALITY CARE IN PUBLIC MENTAL HEALTH PROGRAMS

Stuart L. Keill, M.D.
John A. Talbott, M.D.

The problems of public mental facilities have received widespread lay and professional criticism for many years. Most critics have focused on the failures in administration, leadership, funding, etc., to explain the acknowledged deficiencies. We, however, believe it may be useful to use a systems approach to the problem, and having made this decision selected the metaphor of the filter and filtration process as a vehicle for discussion.*

A filtration bed is defined as "a bed of sand or gravel for filtering water." A broader definition of a filter describes it as

*The concept of filtering patients at the local center so that the least desirable clinical problems go to public facilities is well know.[2,3,4] While this filtering process has changed over the last decade, certain patients continue to be selected for treatment and certain other patients transferred elsewhere.

a "porous mass through which fluid passes while matter in suspension is separated out."[1]

This contribution will describe the functioning of certain public institutions in terms of the effect that a porous filtration process would have on the symbiotic relationship between the organization and its staff. The report is based on the authors' observation of the activities and interviews with the staffs of twelve institutions over the past five years. Eight of the institutions are state psychiatric facilities and four, municipal psychiatric facilities. Biographical sketches or characteristic psychiatrists who work in these facilities and who are affected by them are described. Some details have been deliberately blurred in order to protect the identity of the individuals and the facilities.

THE FILTRATION PROCESS

There are four discernible stages in the Filtration Process:

Stage 1: New Horizons—Shiny Filter

A new program is created either in a previously unserved area or as a replacement for a previously abandoned program. There is considerable enthusiasm on the part of the staff, community leaders, and the media for the inauguration of this new program. It is often described as "a new horizon in mental health, a symbol of a breakthrough," etc. Because of the drama and the general support, an enthusiastic staff is recruited by taking some of the most qualified personnel from other parts of the mental health system and infusing them into the new program. This stage usually consists of two substages: one in which the staff initially plans, then becomes used to the new facility, and finally prepares for the actual treatment of patients; and the second, when the patients begin to be treated at the facility and returned to the community. At this point, morale is high, in spite of possible salary differences with other facilities.[5]

Stage 2: Stabilization—Clean Filter

This state inevitably follows Stage 1 and usually begins approximately two years after the first patients and clients have been seen. There is a slight diminution of the early enthusiasm as the staff becomes familiar to the community, newspapers, etc. as they become frustrated with some of the patients with more difficult problems and interpersonal difficulties begin to emerge. At this stage ordinary staff turnover occurs.[6]

Some of the superior psychiatrists who were attracted to the program initially have begun to leave the program, often because they are upwardly mobile and are recruited by other programs or because they have encountered difficulties with some of their other superior colleagues.[7] In contrast, the least effective staff are not sought by other facilities, tend to be less active, do not seek other employment,[8] and unless they get into serious difficulty, remain in the facility. They are inactive and uncreative and even at this stage, may begin to have a dystonic effect on the program and on their colleagues.

Stage 3: Progressive Stagnation—Advanced Clogging

This stage carries serious prognostic implications. The enthusiasm seen in the earlier stages has seriously deteriorated and may even disappear. Outstanding staff members have either moved on to better pay or more challenging situations, or they have isolated themselves to maintain their integrity within the program. The result is a negligible effect on less effective colleagues. A vicious cycle begins; the image of the program begins to deteriorate; the portion of positions filled with inferior staff increases;[9,10] the morale of the average psychiatrist begins to suffer severely, decreasing his or her effectiveness and motivation; there is less interest by public and the professional groups outside the facility in promoting adequate public support in salaries, of physical plants, etc. This in turn continues to make difficult recruitment of adequate staff;[11,12,13,14,15,16] and the cycle goes on. As the poorer staff continue to stay on and the better staff continue to leave, the proportion of staff items filled by inadequate staff may approach 100 per cent.

Usually these changes, like carcinoma of the lung, remain outside of the awareness of the staff and of the public until too late.[17] (Paradoxically, funding bodies unfamiliar with the details of the program may point to a low turnover of personnel as an indication of good morale, which diminishes their interest in improving the quality of the working situation and the quality of the staff.)

At this point, the health of the patient program is critical, although still reversible. The condition, with little change, may continue for years outside the awareness of the public. There is a vague sense among professionals and local government facilities that the programs are of low quality and inefficient, but they are often tolerated, supported by such comments as, "What can you do or expect?" Occasionally, an outside crisis such as decreasing tax base, loss of staff or a key staff person, may accelerate the deterioration of the program.

On the other hand, the condition may be reversed through heroic therapeutic intervention from the outside. Such intervention may take various forms: (a) It may be the result of the appointment of a new executive through the ordinary process of senior staff turnover. He invariably encounters serious resistance both conscious and unconscious. (b) It may be the result of the interest of a nearby university in finding a suitable clinical campus for their academic program through affiliation. (c) It may be through the interest of a candidate for political office who wishes to make a cause célèbre either to maintain himself in office or to sweep him into office on the crest of the wave of public shock.* (d) It may be the result of a timely and well-organized protest by consumer or community groups who express a conscientious concern about the quality of care provided to their neighbors or families.

Attempts by a new leader to clean the filter are usually

*A variant of this particular device is when the individual is not a political figure but a member of the media who wishes to enhance his repertorial career.

complicated by a nonspecific resistance on the part of the staff toward any change. This kind of resistance, familiar to all those in organizations and analytic practice, is due to a combination of factors: (a) an inability by the individual to accept the fact that he is a participant in or even a supporter of a wasteful and inhumane system; and (b) a somewhat more conscious but understandably human defense against the threat to the inadequately performing professional of being measured in a system in which excellence is required.

Successful and heroic therapeutic interventions occur infrequently at Stage 3, and the next step is inevitably a crisis heralding Stage 4. The crisis may take the form of a shocking event, such as an epidemic, a fire, a staff scandal, or the death of a patient.

Stage 4: Moribund—Obstructed Filter

The death of the facility occurs when both the spirit (or soul) of the program and the body stop functioning. Black's Law Dictionary[18] defines death as "a total stoppage of the circulation of the blood and a cessation of the functions consequent thereon." Theologically speaking, there may be a reincarnation in which the body or skeleton of the institution becomes another facility, such as a large nursing home, an intermediate care facility, or a home for the aged. The soul of the program is salvaged by a mass transfer of the clientele to the other facility, which is usually in Stage 2 or 3. If it is to a facility in Stage 3, it tends to hasten the death of that facility through filter overload. A greater tragedy results when the patients are transferred en masse to a facility in Stage 2, which still has a bright reputation. This may be the key factor in pushing the Stage 2 facility into a Stage 3 category, and the process of recycling continues.[5,17,19]

At times, narcissism leads to literal though of course futile attempts at resurrection. Two of the twelve facilities (not surprisingly the two largest of the twelve) had—in the eyes of all knowledgeable professionals—existed at the Stage 4 level for some time. Recently a coalition of an ambitious governor, willing to sacrifice the effectiveness of his own commissioner; some local legislators; an energetic and articulate, if misguided, body of community consumer representatives; and some representatives of the media, forced tens of millions of dollars, within the course of a few months, into two of the deceased (Stage 4) organizations.*

THE PSYCHIATRISTS IN THE SYSTEM

Assuming all categories of psychiatrists enter the filter system, one can separate them into three categories:

Category 1: The Inadequate Psychiatrist

This person generally has had a mediocre experience in medical school, internship, and residency training, and may often have taken his training in mediocre facilities either in the U.S. or abroad. He is unable to innovate and uninterested in the innovation process. He avoids professional stimuli and of necessity accepts jobs at low salary levels. Because of the civil service systems found in most public facilities, this individual, short of a catastrophe, remains secure in his job.

Case: Dr. J. B. attended medical school following World War II in a Grade B midwestern school. With some difficulty he completed his training in five years and took an internship in a small community hospital in New York State. After three unsuccessful years in private practice as a general practitioner, he took a job as a resident psychiatrist at a rural state psychiatric facility, which he completed in three years without any obvious difficulty. He remained as a junior psychiatrist on the staff for five years until at the instigation of his wife he arranged

*This, tragically, was at the expense of other state programs at the Stage 1 and Stage 2 level, as well as programs outside the system that had been functioning relatively well.

to be transferred to a similar position at a Stage 3 psychiatric facility in New York City. He has not attended a psychiatric meeting since 1968; had never taken the boards; is not a member of the APA; he does admit to reading some of the advertising material on drugs left by the drug company representatives, although he denies that they affect his treatment of patients. He is considered to be a representative member of the middle management of the state facility. His activities generally consist of signing orders, writing prescriptions, and following recommendations of the senior nurse in the unit to which he is assigned. The director of his hospital describes him as a dull, rather schizoid, individual who has never got into any major difficulties, although he is generally disliked by both the nursing and social service personnel with whom he works. The director describes him as no better and no worse than 75 per cent of his staff. "I couldn't get rid of him if I wanted to, but even if I could, who would replace him?"

Category 2: The Average Psychiatrist

This psychiatrist, although occasionally endowed with superior intelligence, is not particularly creative. His activity is largely determined by the professional milieu and his colleagues. He's usually successful in the boards on the first or second try, but may fail to develop further. He attends professional meetings, but ordinarily sees them as primarily social or recreational occasions that are "tax deductible." In a stimulating facility, this psychiatrist, challenged by consistent high expectations by his supervisor, may provide the foundation of the organization with good quality services. He carries out his activities under the guidance of an interested superior and on occasion may even go "beyond the call of duty." In a pathologic or defective organization, his productivity gradually tends to decrease. The programs for which he is responsible deteriorate, and he lacks insight ordinarily into the deteriorating process.[20] This latter process is usually reversible if the environment or the supervision is modified.

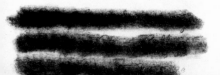

Average psychiatrist in a Stage II facility:

Case: Dr. A. R. graduated from a Class A medical school in Pennsylvania in the early 1950s. He interned at an affiliated university hospital, and then began a residency at a state psychiatric hospital affiliated rather loosely with the general hospital. Following the completion of his residency he took a junior staff position at the hospital and has continued on the staff since. In the interim, nine years after completion of his residency, he passed his boards on the second try. He progressed through the civil service system successfully but without any particular distinction so that at the present time he is one of the senior administrative psychiatrists at the facility. The director of the facility is concerned with teaching programs, many of which take place outside the hospital. Dr. A. R. responded to this stimuli by conducting a rather unexciting but consistent clinical conference; making regular checks of the quality of the charts on patients in the hospital; and attending all autopsies. He attends the APA meetings on alternate years, and carries on a small private practice after hours, which he finds interesting and financially rewarding.

Average psychiatrist in a Stage III facility:

Case: Dr. N. R. attended a Grade A medical school in New York City, graduated in the middle of his class, interned at a small general hospital in the same borough as his medical school, and took his residency at a municipal hospital in New York City, where he was considered an average resident. Following the completion of his residency, he was given a part-time job on the staff of the hospital and began to build a private practice, which was reasonably successful. After a year of this, however, he moved to an area outside the city where he took a job at a state facility as a junior staff person. He has remained on the staff at essentially a middle-grade level in this public facility for the past ten years. After one rather passive and unsuccessful attempt to complete the boards, he became resigned to practicing without them. Since there was little consensus interest in clinical conferences at the facility where he worked, he continued to perform his clinical activities in a rather lackadaisical fashion. On occasion he would pass off his responsibilities to others and this seemed to have excited no reaction either from his superiors or from his colleagues. He told one of the authors, "It's all rather fruitless to knock yourself out; it doesn't pay off, and nobody notices anyway." He has not attended a psychiatric meeting in years, but he maintains his membership in the APA. Although he has current interest and knowledge of minor medications, useful in some private practices, he expresses no interest or awareness of current treatment techniques for the more serious disorders.

Category 3: The Superior Psychiatrist

(The reader by the very fact of reading this chapter unquestionably falls in this category.) This individual is generally of superior intelligence and has demonstrated consistent and considerable success in medical school, internship, and residency. He tends to be particularly interested in teaching and in professional activities and often in contributions to professional journals (20).

Case: Dr. G. G. graduated in the upper third of his class from one of the leading medical schools in the New York City metropolitan area. He took his internship at a university hospital. His first two years of residency training were completed at another university hospital. Because of his family responsibilities, he completed his third year in a public service facility outside the area and stayed on at that hospital in a junior staff position while starting a small practice. Eight months after his arrival at the hospital, an older colleague who was the chief of one of the units became ill and an attempt was made to secure a volunteer from within to replace him. Since none of the senior staff at this Stage 3 facility wished to "take on anything new," Dr. G. G. was asked to assume the direction of the unit. Within three months, the unit developed a somewhat more active patient program, although there were serious complaints from the older staff about some of his "crazy new ideas." However, a new enthusiasm began to appear among the staff. Two years following the completion of his residency, he successfully passed his boards on the initial attempt. By this time he was having difficulties with the director of the hospital, to whom he had on several occasions complained of lack of support for the necessary new programs in his unit. One year following completion of his boards, he accepted a job in a university program that carried a modest increase in salary but would have been considered comparable to one of the Stage 1 programs.

Case: Dr. M. K. completed medical school in the early 1960s at a major school where he graduated in the upper third of his class. He completed an internship at a major general hospital in the Midwest where he took a university residency for three years. On completion of this he returned to accept a position as a junior psychiatrist at a facility entering Stage 3. As soon as he was eligible to take the boards, he did so and completed them successfully. On this basis, since many of the board psychiatrists at this facility accepted had positions elsewhere, he was asked to take charge of the residency program. He was active in the local district branch of the APA, was the author of several papers, pursued a fairly active private practice, began to become increasingly discouraged about the service aspects in which he worked, and gradually became more and more isolated from his staff colleagues. As a result of this, he became increasingly protective of the resident staff who idolized him, and who, in many cases because of their contact with him, had a superior working knowledge in psychiatry to the senior staff psychiatrists in the hospital. His evident concern with quality increasingly turned the other psychiatrists against him, which furthered the walling-off process between him and the rest of the organization. At this writing it is now becoming increasingly difficult for this facility to attract good residents since the quality teaching at the facility is almost entirely limited to the efforts of this physician.

The authors have not cited instances of a superior psychiatrist in a superior facility since the kind of problems this relationship presents does not relate to this discussion.

THE PRESCREENING PROCESS

In a discussion of the filtration effect on staff competence, there is of course a prescreening process.[20,21,22] There is a well-documented effect on the recruitment of staff prior to the more obvious filtration process described. Gurel[22] noted that while only 20 per cent of U.S. medical school graduates seeking full-time psychiatric staff positions accept jobs in the so-called public facilities, 57 per cent of foreign graduates accepting positions do so in public facilities. Of the full-time staff in nonpublic facilities, 65 per cent have been certified by the American Board of Psychiatry and Neurology, while in the public facilities, only 32 per cent have been. West[23] commented on the good image of psychiatric services in the "medical community" contrasted with what was described as a bad image some years ago. This good image, however, pertained to the university general hospital setting where there is day-to-day contact and cross-fertilization with other members of the medical community.

As a result of this prefiltration process, those psychiatrists who are unable to meet the standards of the quality facilities and those who have difficulties maintaining a successful private practice tend to migrate toward facilities where the salary scale is low and where the image in the professional community tends to be poor. In New York State these generally are the state psychiatric centers. Municipal hospitals are somewhat less affected by this system because they are generally affiliated with medical schools and are usually part of general hospitals despite the fact that they, like the state facilities, are hampered by a low salary scale and the civil service system. Even here, however, there are various courses of facility development, and examples of this typology are noted in the four municipal hospitals studied by the authors. One hospital developed a two-class system of services in which there was a small quality program where most of the teaching took place and where the type of patient admitted was carefully selective. At the same time at the same facility, the majority of patients were served in a massive unit where the staff and the quality of care was similar to the characteristics described in the state facilities. A second municipal facility also affiliated with a major university was smaller, had a relatively good teaching program and fairly good staff morale, but was unable to provide the quantity of services that the system demanded. The result was that patients were consistently shunted elsewhere. A third example was a facility that consistently carried out a very large patient-care job but of consistently low quality.

DISCUSSION

Following the study of the life cycle of 12 facilities, and the types of psychiatrists at these facilities, it is evident that they have a powerful effect on one another.[24,25,26] Unfortunately, the effect is destructive symbiosis in most cases. These facilities in the public section even when started with a bright prognosis and considerable enthusiasm, inevitably begin to collect inferior professionals. Early in the history of an organization, an appropriate balance of superior and average professionals are attracted in spite of some of the disadvantages of the system.* Shortly thereafter problems begin to develop. As with Gresham's Law, the number of poor psychiatrists increases while the number of good psychiatrists decreases. The alert executive in an organization entering this stage is constantly attentive to the above development and "cleans the filter" through staff reassignment, salesmanship, seduction, and staff education.** He rewards professional growth, and through a filter-cleaning

*Similar to the effect noted in Macarov's study of a kibbutz.[30]
**Gerard [9] has said, "for learning to take place, the student must carry on the behavior to be learned and find it satisfactory." Others agree.[10,11]

process, strives to maintain the functioning of the organization at the late Stage 1/early Stage 2 period.[27,28]

Without this, fewer good psychiatrists are attracted to the organization. Those who do either leave shortly or isolate themselves within the organization. The inferior professionals continue to be attracted since they have difficulty surviving elsewhere, but unlike the superior ones, they tend to remain. The program begins to deteriorate, the performance of the average psychiatrist also deteriorates, the image of the facility declines, the morale worsens, and the services become inadequate.[29] Finally it reaches, in Reiss's terms "the point of staff and patient hopelessness when the hospital is in the process of agonal dissolution."[5]

Since each of these facilities is part of the large statewide system, one could predict the impact of many clogged filters on the larger system. In 1966 a new commissioner was appointed to head the New York State Department of Mental Hygiene. Vigorous efforts to clean the filters took place, including major new concepts, the importation of a variety of talented staff from outside the system, and repeated injections of major new expenditures into the system. For a time it appeared as if these attempts might be successful, in spite of a major progressive accumulation of problems, low morale, chronicity of patients, obsolete institutions, poor image, and considerable internal institutional resistance to change. By late 1973, however, it was apparent that in spite of the best intentions and all of the money, it was a losing battle. At least 80 per cent of the facilities in the state system at the time could be categorized as being in Stage 3.

While most people receiving psychiatric treatment were receiving it from facilities other than the state facilities, 90 per cent of the total state expenditures for mental health went into the maintenance of what was essentially a clogged filter system. Shortly, the energies of the commissioner and his key staff were absorbed in answering increasingly frequent attacks from the public, the news media, and consumer groups. The final outcome was a change in state administration with the departure of most of the senior departmental personnel. The new state executive branch appeared to assume that enough attention, enough money, and three distinguished leaders in the central office could restore the dead facilities to life and resuscitate the system. To date the deterioration continues.

In many cases, genuine damage to the effectiveness of some superior personnel within the system occurred. This in turn has led to increased difficulty in recruiting effective and managerial staff with quality credentials, thus accelerating the downward spiral. One could extend the concepts described to other public service settings where there have been major administrative problems, such as the prison and judicial systems, the New York City public school system, and the nursing home situation.

CONCLUSION

On the basis of a combined experience in one large state where the attempt to produce and maintain quality in a large system failed in spite of tremendous number of talented personnel and excessive funding, we doubt that it is possible for a large centralized system to clean the filter periodically and thereby preserve efficient and effective programming.

There is little hope that public facilities will be able to compete for staff with the private sector financially. Some alert executives at localized facilities may be successful in improving programs and maintaining the morale of the professional staff. There is more day-to-day contact of the providers and the consumers, and there is a somewhat closer accountability of the branches of government to the taxpayer. This, combined with alert attention to the filtration process (routinely cleansing or replacement of the filter at least every two years), may make it possible to continue quality care still affordable by a public service system.[27,28,31] It has been successful so far in three of the facilities studied by the authors. However, it requires constant vigilance and most surely an energetic enthusiasm bordering on the hypomanic. It also requires an alliance with at least one power base outside the system, i.e., a sympathetic media contact, a consumer group, or a strong political figure. Those in the position of executive authority at local human service facilities should see filter cleaning in a locally administered program as a challenge and a hope. Given the inevitability of changes in our mental health system, it may be the only hope.

SUMMARY

The authors have described administrative problems and solutions in public mental health programs as seen via the metaphor of a "filtration bed." Four stages in the life cycle of such programs were described from the beginning of a new program to the terminal phase, using filter bed "titles." Focusing on the psychiatrists, as one integral segment of these programs, the effect of program quality on good, average, and poor psychiatrists was noted.

The authors concluded that energetic and continued attention to "cleaning the filter" in local programs may maintain the quality of a good program, utilize effectively the potential of the staff, and even affect the larger system of which the local facilities are a part.

REFERENCES

1. *Webster's New Collegiate Dictionary,* Springfield, Mass.: Merriam, 1976.

2. Gervais, R., et al.: "Changing Patterns of Psychiatric Inpatient Care in a University General Hospital." *American Journal of Psychiatry* 132:12, 1272–1275, December 1975.

3. Feigelson, E.: Personal communications.

4. Ozarin, L. D., & Taube, C. A.: "Psychiatric Inpatients: Who, Where and Future." *American Journal of Psychiatry* 121:98–101, 1974.

5. Reiss, D., et al.: "Personal Needs, Values and Technical Preferences in the Psychiatric Hospital." *Archives of General Psychiatry* 33 (7):795–804, 1976.

6. Spillane, R.: "Instrinsic and Extrinsic Job Satisfaction and Labour Turnover: A Questionnaire Study of Australian Managers." *Occupational Psychology* (London) 47 (1–2):71–74, 1973.

7. Jenning, E.: "Mobiocentric Man." *Psychology Today,* June 1970.

8. Bowman, M. P.: "Management-1: Individual and Personality Growth." *Nursing Times* (London), 71(26):1022–1023, 1975.

9. Gerard, R.: Conference on "Psychiatric Education in Medical Schools" American Psychiatric Association, Washington, D.C., 1969.

10. Tyler, R. W.: Opening Address and Charge to the Conference: Teaching Psychiatry in Medical School. Published by the Preparatory Commission for the Conference on Psychiatry and Medical Education, American Psychiatric Association, Washington, D. C., 1969.

11. Hines, G. H.: "Cross-Cultural Differences in Two-Factor Motivation Theory." *Journal of Applied Psychology,* 58(3):375–377, 1973.

12. Karp, H. B., & Nickson, J. W., Jr.: "Motivator-Hygiene Deprivation as a Predictor of Job Turnover." *Personnel Psychology,* 26(3): 377–384, 1973.

13. Gordon, M. E., Pryor, N. M., & Harris, B. V.: An Examination of Scaling Bias in Herzberg's Theory of Job Satisfaction. Organizational Behavior and Human Performance, 11(1):106–121, 1974.

14. Reynolds, M.: "Perceptual Defense and Herzberg's Methodology: A Basis for Understanding Commitment to Work." *Interpersonal Development* (Basel), 4(3): 170–176, 1974.

15. Giovannini, P. C.: *A Study of the Interaction Between Job Satisfaction, Job Involvement, and Job Performance.* (Ph.D. dissertation). Ann Arbor, Mich.: Disserattion Abstracts International 1974.

16. Rogers, K.: State Mental Hospitals: An Organizational Analysis. Administration in Mental Health, Fall 1975.

17. Greenblatt, M., & Glazier, E.: "The Phasing Out of Mental Hospitals in the United States." *American Journal of Psychiatry,* 132:11 1135–1140, November 1975.

18. *Black's Law Dictionary.* St. Paul, Minn.: West Publishing Co., 4th ed, 1968.

19. Cressey D. R.: "A Confrontation of Violent Dynamics." *International Psychiatry,* 10(3): 109–130, 1972.

20. National Institute of Mental Health: *Staffing of Mental Health Facilities.* U.S. 1972 Department of Health, Education, and Welfare Publication #ADM74-28. Washington, D. C.: U.S. Government Printing Office, 1972.

21. Hammatt, V. B. O., & Spivack G.: "What residents do after graduation." *Archives of General Psychiatry,* 33:415–416, 1976.

22. Gurel, L.: *A Survey of Academic Resources in Psychiatric Residency Training.* Published by Division of Manpower Research and Development, American Psychiatric Association, Washington, D. C., June 1973.

23. West N. D., & Walsh M. A.: "Psychiatry's image today: results of an attitudinal survey." American Journal of Psychiatry 132:12, 1218–1219, December 1975.

24. McGregor D.: "The Human Side of Enterprise" in Management of Human Resources, Pigors, J. W., et al., eds., New York: McGraw Hill 2nd ed., 1969.

25. Stanton A., & Schwartz, M.: *The Mental Hospital,* New York: Basic Books, 1954.

26. Barton, W. E.: *Administration in Psychiatry.* Springfield, Ill.: Charles C. Thomas, 1962.

27. Goldman, H.: "Conflict, Competition and Coexistence: The Mental Hospital as Parallel Health and Welfare Systems." *American Journal of Orthopsychiatry,* 47, 60–65, January 1977.

28. Elster, R. S., Githens, W. H., & Senger, J. D.: "Need structure analysis of organizational policies." Psychological Reports 37(3):1123–1131, 1975.

29. Goffman, E.: *Asylum.* Garden City, N.Y.: Doubleday, 1961.

30. Macarov, D.: "Work patterns and satisfactions in an Israeli kibbutz: A test of the Herzberg hypothesis." *Personnel Psychology,* 25(3):483–493, 1972.

31. Feldman, S DPA: *The Administration of Mental Health Services.* Springfield, Ill: Charles C Thomas, 1973.

Chapter 6

A TYPOLOGY OF STATE HOSPITAL DIRECTORS

John A. Talbott, M.D.
Stuart L. Keill, M.D.

Introduction

There has been little attention in the literature to the directors of state mental health facilities, despite the fact that each year they are responsible for the care provided in over 25 percent of the inpatient mental health care episodes.[1] It is our intention in this chapter to correct this neglect by proposing a typology of directors of state facilities, drawing upon our combined 35 years experience in the New York State Department of Mental Hygiene, beginning as psychiatric residents and culminating as state mental hospital director and state regional commissioner, respectively.

Of necessity, any typology depends on the clearest and most memorable examples to identify specific types and subtypes. Our typology is no exception. The examples cited, therefore, tend to be obvious, colorful, and vaguely pejorative. But it must be remembered that we too are members of the group

Illustrations by Miska Synowiecka.

we are describing and share in the selfsame faults and foibles we describe. We have consciously attempted to sketch caricatures of typical director-types rather than paint more balanced realistic portraits. While relationships between the level of care, administrative style, personality variables, and the director-types we describe may exist in the real world, these are most assuredly not one-to-one correlations. It is out firm conviction that both good and bad directors have good and bad characteristics.

The methodology follows that proposed by Robert Michels in "A Field Guide to Psychiatric Educators in North America."[2] For each director-type we will state a motto or rallying cry that typifies him; describe the type in some detail; give examples of his ego-ideal, goal in life, hero and antihero; enumerate what he reads and believes; state his views on mental illness and his priorities on service, teaching, and research; and specify his administrative and leadership styles and preferential table of organization. While we do not refer to our types and subtypes in traditional administrative terms, we are indebted to such authors as Max Weber, Rensis Likert, and Robert Blake and Jane Mouton.[3,4,5]

TYPOLOGY

1. The Saintly Director (Figure 1)

Our first director-type is that of the Saintly Director, whose motto is "Try to do as I do." He or she is usually committed, hardworking, passionate, persuasive, and knowledgeable and believes that good intentions conquer all. His ego-ideal is the individual who is able to overcome overwhelming adversity through apostolic words and a saintly demeanor, and his goal in life is to inspire one or two disciples to follow his path to righteousness. His hero is a combination of Florence Nightingale and Marie Curie and his antihero is the Cynical Director, to be discussed later.

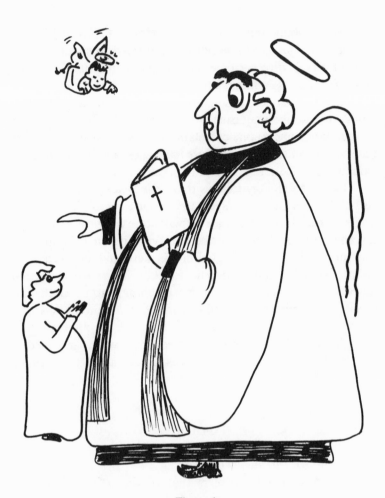

Figure 1

He reads the current psychiatric literature and believes in the goodness of service to his fellow man. His views on treating the mentally ill are that, given the proper tools, the unselfish right people and a loving attitude, he can do the job. For him, service is primary; training is a far-distant second priority; and research is not in contention in his list of interests.

His leadership style is to lead by example and his administrative style is overcommitment, underdelegation and guilt-producing exhortation. His table of organization resembles that of a Boy Scout troop where the highest positions go to the super-aspirant, most committed, and hardest working.

Since the Saintly Director relies on his personal commitment and example to inspire others, he falls prey to disorganization, unrealistic idealism and overvaluation of hours worked and numbers of patients seen rather than programmatic or therapeutic impact. However, on balance, despite such pitfalls, he or she tends to be an examplary, if somewhat annoying, director.

2. The Renaissance Director (Figure 2)

Our second category is the Renaissance Director, whose motto is "Judge me by my publications." This type tends to be bright, imaginative, narcissistic, exhibitionistic, and power-hungry. He does a great deal of "thinking" around the office. He is perpetually involved in areas that are not the primary mission of the hospital, e.g. public relations, conceptual issues, the process of change itself, and departmental, university, or professional politics. His ego-ideal and goal is to make the biggest impact possible. His hero is Oliver Wendell Holmes or Paul de Kruif and his antihero Thomas Szasz.

He reads widely—*Science, Dedalus, Scientific American, Nature* and books written by sociologists and anthropologists. He believes in his own rightness and thinks he has the answers to the problems of mental illness. As such, he usually perceives the Department of Mental Hygiene as obstructing his initiative

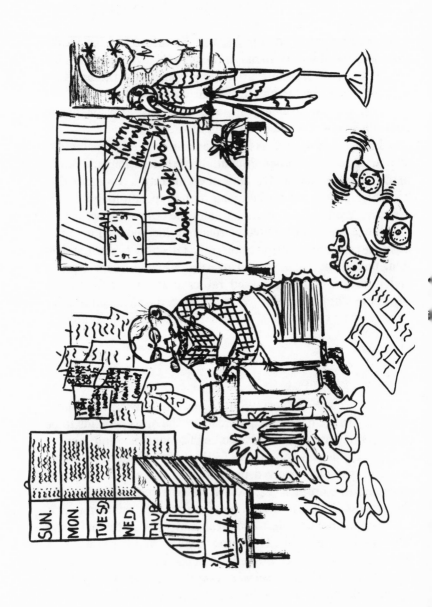

in solving the great problems of our time. Research for him is primary, training a close second, and service a distant third.

His leadership style is to lead by passionate exhortation and his administrative style leans heavily on changing the organization according to his personal standards and relying on subordinates to carry out his proclamations while he acquires new ideas, new data, and new programs. Thus, his table of organization reflects the thrust of his cherished notions, and information tends to flow only downwards.

The pitfalls of this director are that he often becomes emotionally detached, may become an absentee innovator, and frequently gets into trouble with the system and his superiors because of his devotion to other interests and benign neglect of his clinical responsibilities. However, his immediate subordinates usually revere him and his powerful presence usually moves the organization in positive directions.

3. Lunatic Fringe (Figure 3)

This director is essentially a subtype of the Renaissance Director—gone amok. This director's motto is "What crusade shall we promote this week?" This subtype has all the characteristics of the above, compounded by charisma, egocentricity, and egotism. This director's ego-ideal and goals in life can only be inferred from his acts, but seem idiosyncratic and hidden from those around him. His hero is a combination of John Brown, Frantz Fanon, and T. E. Lawrence and his antihero any other member of the lunatic fringe.

He reads the *Village Voice, Screw,* Albert Einstein, and The Book of Book or some other piece of "in" Sufi literature. He believes even more fervently than the Renaissance Director that he has the answers, and views the Department of Mental Hygiene as a hostile opponent in his crusade for curing mental illness. Service, research, and teaching are all equally unimportant since only the current crusade has priority.

This director's leadership style is haranguing; rage and

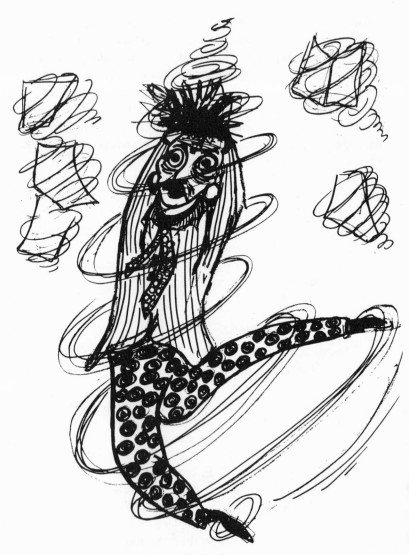

Figure 3

ecstasy and his administrative style depends on a cadre of high-ly-trusted guerrilla fighters who carry on the crusade while it lasts. The table of organization is forever changing, a kaleido-scopic phenomenon.

The pitfalls of this style are inherent in its description. Change is embraced in panicky ways, there is organizational chaos and diffusion of energy as crusades proliferate and re-place each other, and the director at extreme points is viewed as crazy or paranoid and engages in spirited dancing (not unlike an ecstatic whirling dervish). About the only good thing that can be said about him is that life is never dull and that as a by-product of one or another crusade, some patients are inevita-bly helped.

4. Grandfather (Figure 4)

Our fourth type is the Grandfather Director whose motto is "You know I know best, now just do as I say." These direc-tors are parental in all their activities, acting as fathers, moth-ers, or nursemaids to the staff and patients. The hospital is viewed as one big family with the overriding task to keep the family intact and happy. Inquiries from above are seen as intru-sions into the family's business and problems are handled by disciplining the bad boys. Here the ego-ideal is that of a grand-parent and the goal in life is to maintain a warm family. This director's hero is Rose Kennedy or Mary Lasker and his an-tihero is James Dean or Abbie Hoffman.

He reads the Book of the Month, *Reader's Digest,* and the *Civil Service Leader* and believes what his family believes. He pays lip service to current concepts in the treatment of the mentally ill, knowing secretly that all that really counts is warm familial love. Contentment is seen as progress, and the bureau-cracy is fine so long as it stays away from the family's affairs. Service is his only priority.

The director's leadership style is thoroughly parental, leading the family like a mother or father, and his or her admin-

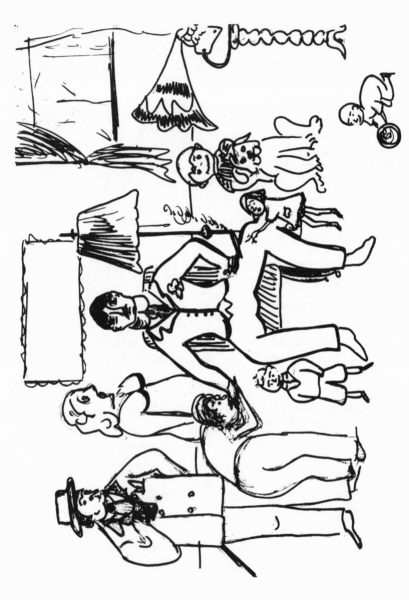

Figure 4

istrative style depends heavily on informal networks, personal loyalty, and charismatic qualities. He is cautious, playing his cards close to his vest, and he frequently uses Machiavellian techniques to play off parts of the organization against each other in order to maintain control of the clan.

Since the director's personal image and his staff's satisfaction are important and interwined, the pitfalls of this style involve total abrogation of duty in performing any tasks, and the hiring and protection of real and acquired family members. On the other hand, as long as father's will is done, there is peace and quiet and the family is the ideal place to be.

5. The Old Guard Director (Figure 5)

Our next category of typical director is the Old Guard Director whose motto is "The good old days were better" and "We'd better go slow now, fellas." This director clings to the past, fights change as if it represents death, frequently gives in to futility, and devotes the majority of his time to protecting his flanks. When in doubt he (1) does nothing, (2) calls Albany, or (3) goes by the book. His ego-ideal is the revered psychiatrist-administrator of yore and his sole goal in life is returning to the halcyon days. His heros are Benjamin Rush and Adolf Meyer and his antihero the president of the Federation of Parents' Organizations.

He reads history, literature, and Henderson and Gillespie, and believes that there's nothing new in psychiatry, so why try to change things. Progress is seen as interesting but unimportant, and bureaucracy is felt to be comforting as long as it supports the status quo. Among service, training, and research, training is thought be all-important and while there is little interest in service, interest in research is nonexistent. Survival and the maintenance of perquisites, such as laundry, mail service, food, and a chauffered car, are the only truly important things.

His leadership style is apologetically authoritarian, and his

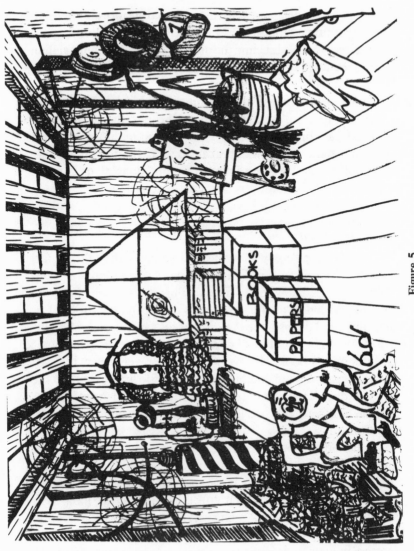

Figure 5

administrative style places maximum stress on rules and regulations, paper procedures, keeping out of trouble, monitoring and disciplining, and balancing authority, responsibility, delegation, and accountability to conform to some long-lost idealized administrative formula. His table of organization stresses traditional line authority, and persons move up the chart according to seniority and ability to breathe rather than because of merit, excellence, and performance.

The pitfalls of this director are complete paralysis, depression, adaption to the role of cynical victim, and lack of interest in anything but staying alive, personally and organizationally. On the other hand, some are realistic and reasonable and fit ideally into a completely bureaucratic structure with all its deficiencies.

6. The Uninvolved Director (Figure 6)

The next category is that of the Uninvolved Director whose motto is "It's not bad because it never happened." This director-type believes that the hospital functions efficiently, because he hasn't the foggiest notion what's going on. He may be inconsistent or arrogant but above all he is not aware or affected by the real state of affairs, because he's not involved, either because he's absent from his job, stupid, or insensitive. He has no ego-ideal and his goal in life is acceptance by his subordinates. He has no hero or antihero because he's not sure what route he's on.

He reads irrespective of the media or contents, and it matters little because nothing impresses or interests him anyway. And he believes that everything is good whether it's treatment, progress, or the bureaucracy. He has no preference for service, training, or research because it doesn't really matter.

His style of leadership is the maintenance of one or two areas of interest and delegation of all other items. His administrative style, therefore, relies heavily on overdelegation and abrogation of responsibility. His table of organization depends

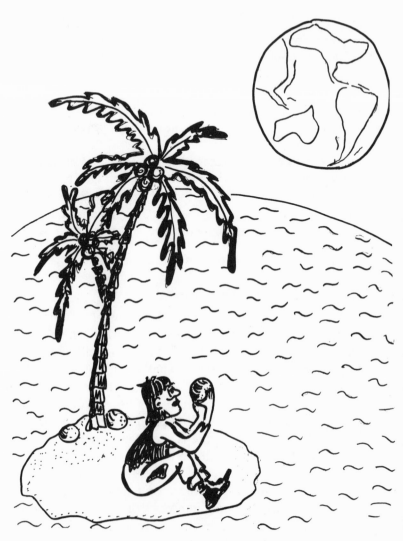

Figure 6

always and excessively on middle management and thus may be top-heavy. Regardless of the formal organization, however, the informal structure either deals with business (and may do so extremely well) or the organization is a complete disaster.

The pitfalls of this type of director involve the issue of delegation. If middle management tries to seek direction or is incapable of running the show, the hospital will falter. However, if the top subordinates can manage effectively, the hospital may run well, and the director proceeds merrily through life oblivious to the reality of the complex environment.

7. The Cynical Director (Figure 7)

Our last category is that of the Cynical Director whose motto is "What have those fools in Albany done now?" This director is a chronic complainer, who while bitter and cynical, is "always right." To him, all trouble emanates from above, and he doesn't do much, despite his often impressive intelligence, because he enjoys demonstrating how others are screwing up, more than testing out his own ideas. His ego-ideal is demonstrating the foolishness of others, and his goal in life to expose their inadequacy. He professes, however, the goal of achieving peace and quiet. His hero is the Last Angry Man and his antihero the Saintly Director.

He reads widely to buttress his litany of complaints and while he believes in little, he in convinced that any failures come from without. He views attempts to treat mental illness as all well in theory but impossible to implement. He is skeptical of achieving progress and assumes that the bureaucracy can only make things worse. He has no preference for service, teaching, or research since all these are futile endeavors.

His leadership style is one of abrogation, he's too busy taking care of important matters—such as pets, restrooms, elevators, or parking spaces—to worry about such mundane matters as the hospital. His administrative style is an unstated delegation of almost all tasks to others, who since they are

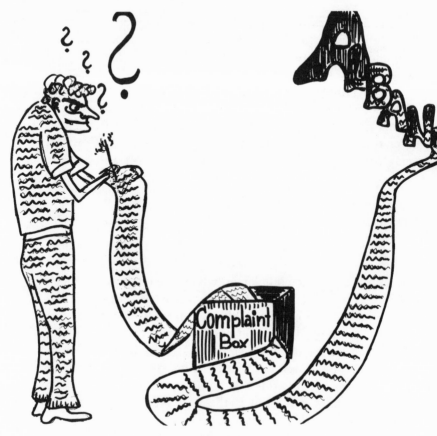

Figure 7

unaware of such delegation, tend to do little. His table of organization looks fine on paper but can meet few basic needs.

The one redeeming quality of this type is his humor and wit. For while his organization may founder, and his patient care stagnate, he offers his troops ample reasons for their plight, couched in devastating and often accurate terms.

DISCUSSION

If our typology (with apologies to the real characters) approximates the truth, one would expect major differences in the hospitals administered by the seven different types of directors described above. It is our experience, however, that, despite our allusions to well-run versus poorly run organizations, there are no clear correlations between these director-types and the success or failure of their organizations. Certainly there are differences in morale, innovation, and where human energies are spent. But in the final analysis, as recorders and close observers, we wind up adjacent to the cynicism or at least the skepticism of the last mentioned director-type.

Why is this? We believe there are multiple factors, most of which are in fact out of the director's control. These include: the existing rules and regulations, the civil service system, the budgetary constraints and inflexibilities, the patient population, the lack of prestige of state service, the difficulty of institutional change in long-standing bureaucratic structure, the overwhelming nature of the public health responsibility inherited by the director, and the type and quality of the lower echelons of staff attracted to and maintained in the hospital.

Not all directors begin as cynical, uninvolved, or lunatic; many start as saintly, renaissance men and women, but develop defenses to deal with the frustration of their jobs. Such defenses may include denial, projection, displacement, insensitivity, retreat, involvement in other activities, cynicism, devotion to self-preservation, or an emphasis on any change or the change process as an end in itself. Others actually leave the field, and resign or move upstairs in the departmental hierarchy.[6] Few survive with continuing energy and commitment to their tasks.

It is interesting that the authors, as well as the directors and administrators with whom we have shard this contribution, tend to see themselves as combining the best features of the saintly, renaissance, Grandfather, and cynical directors, while omitting all the negative features.

Lest the reader assume we are unequivocably condemnatory about state hospital directors, we should state emphatically that there are a number of admirable qualities with which many directors begin their directorships. They are a commitment to service and public psychiatry; intelligence, wit, and training. And, lest the reader assume that our descriptions are applicable only to psychiatrists serving as directors in state facilities, several readers of our earlier drafts assured us that our descriptions are equally valid as descriptions of a variety of administrators, not the least of whom are the academic chairmen of departments of psychiatry.

SUMMARY

We have described seven types of state hospital directors. Our discussion focused on the inevitability of the development of nonproductive defenses and character-styles in most of those who assume leadership positions in state facilities due to a number of factors. We also discuss our observation that there is no correlation between the typology and organizational effectiveness. Our conclusion from this is that it doesn't really matter what type of director is placed in the job, so long as the system, with all its bureaucratic complexities and program responsibilities, is bigger than any of them. We suspect that without good leadership and localized accountability it is very difficult to have both a quality and public mental health system, at least as our departments of mental health are now constituted.

REFERENCES

1. Taube, C. A., & Redick, R. W.: *Provisional Data on Patient Care Episodes in Mental Health Facilities,* 1973, Mental Health Statistical Note. No. 127, National Institute of Mental Health, Washington, D.C., U.S. Department of Health, Education, and Welfare, February 1976.

2. Michels, R. A.: "A Field Guide to Psychiatric Educators in North America." Unpublished paper, November 1970.

3. Blake, R. R., & Mouton, J. S.: *The Managerial Grid.* Houston: Gulf Publishing Co., 1964.

4. Likert, R.: *New Patterns of Management.* New York: McGraw-Hill, 1961.

5. Weber, M.: *The Theory of Social and Economic Organizations.* New York: The Free Press, 1964.

6. Keill, S. L., & Talbott, J. A.: "The Filtration Bed Phenomenon and Its Relation to Staff Competence and Quality Care in Public Mental Health Programs." Chapter 5, this volume.

Chapter 7

THE DEMISE OF A HOSPITAL: DEMOCRATIC–AUTOCRATIC

Robert M. Daly, M.D.

During the first ten years of its existence, a particular state hospital recruited tremendous human resources, utilized the most advanced and proven technical knowledge and fostered both applied and basic research to become one of the leading psychiatric centers in the state. Because of its dynamic approach to mental health service delivery, it was able to expand its original urban catchment area of one-half million to service 1.5 million people with an inpatient census of approximately 600 and an average duration of patient stay of 35 days. It affiliated with a community-conscious medical school, which provided a dynamic superintendent with a superior reputation for teaching, research, service, and administration. Its geographic units were an integrated part of an open system with the comprehensive community-based services. There were no barriers to continuity of care. State, county, and private services flowed into each other in a coordinated fashion. Decision-making, conflict resolution, and policy planning were performed by heterogeneous groups within the total system of care. The superintendent encouraged each unit-system to develop its own homeostasis. As a result, each geographic unit created a unique dynamism in adopting to the needs of its catchment area.

The hospital's regional units were, similarly, responsive to the needs of the total population and, as a result, there developed a maximum security forensic service, a psychiatric geriatric service, an adolescent day service, a cognitive development service, a day care service for young children of schizophrenic mothers, and a long-term rehabilitation service for schizophrenic patients with "the social breakdown syndrome." There were special divisions concentrating on family therapy, group process, and spatial relationships. Besides continuous stimulation of research throughout the hospital, there also existed a controlled psychopharamacological research ward.

In addition to each unit's educating and training its mental health manpower for its own particular purposes, the superintendent with staff from the medical school initiated a new type of community-oriented residency program that became a national model. He also affiliated the hospital with a community college and developed a career ladder leading to an associate degree for the mental health workers.

Professionals of all disciplines were eager to join the staff of this dynamic educational, treatment, and research psychiatric center. In response to a continually changing mental health environment, policy and planning were everyone's responsibility; coordinated and ultimately implemented by the superintendent. New technology, if presented in a rational, well-considered, and enthusiastic manner, was generously tested. It is worth mentioning that despite this expensive staff and technology and high cost per patient day, the cost per patient illness was one of the lowest in the state.

Within two years after a change in leadership almost all of its human assets had vanished or their creativity repressed. This was not caused through any malicious intention of the new superintendent. In fact, he was a gentleman, a scholar, and a prestigious psychiatrist whose only goal was to improve the functioning and the reputation of the hospital. What caused the surprisingly rapid exodus of professional personnel was the change of administrative styles.

In a human service institution, such as a state hospital, a well-organized, highly skilled, creative staff is a much more important element than any quantifiable measurement. Until some scheme is found by which this imponderable of the clinical organization may be assayed and given definite statistical expression, its disappearance is rarely appreciated by central public mental health officials who are delegated to control and evaluate the mental health delivery system.[1] This chapter will attempt to analyze the change in management styles that affected so drastically invaluable human resources. The root cause can be learned by understanding the difference between a duality in leadership types, mutually antagonistic in nature and represented by a proliferation of paired-opposite terms. I refer to the following: democratic–autocratic, participating–hierarchical, mechanic–organic, human relations–scientific management, theory X–theory Y, etc.

THE HOSPITAL AS A SYSTEM

I will start from the obvious premise that the present state psychiatric hospital is a complex organization enmeshed in a dynamic environment and changing conditions, which give rise constantly to fresh problems and unforeseen requirements for action that cannot be broken down or distributed automatically. This is manifested in its new role in regional planning and evaluation, its adjustment to the process of disinstitutionalization and phasing down, its move towards geographic unitization with its concomitant sharing of decision making with the community provider, its transformation from custodial care to therapeutic milieu, its need to comply with multiple regulating and licensing agencies, and finally its emergence as an educational center, developing career ladders for paraprofessionals and training and research for professionals. Amidst all of this turbulence, the state hospital has also had to deal with the new role of the unions, perverted political priorities, patient rights movements, baffling economic problems, the all-enveloping consumer participation, and, last but not least, the entanglements of the legal profession as they pursue their self-imposed holy mandate to eliminate all social evils by legislation and court action.

The state psychiatric hospital is, in reality, a dynamic decision system that must analyze constantly changing current data and integrate it with the overall objectives of the organization. In this regard, it is useful to consider the total hospital organization as a communication network. Realizing that a systems approach to its governance is essential, McDonough and Garrett compare certain major differences between this approach and traditional organizational approaches as follows:[2]

a) Organization emphasizes the design of the organizational structure and then thinks of the communications needed for this structure. (Systems emphasize the design of communications structure and then think of the organization needed to complement this structure.)

b) Organization stresses chain of command, authority, and responsibility. (Systems stress channels of communication, information flow, and decisions.)

c) Organization provides compartments of authority and responsibility. (Systems provide networks between question and answer points.)

THE ORGANIZATIONAL STRUCTURE

Therefore, my second premise is that the traditional bureaucracy, which has served organizations so well in the past, cannot survive as the dominant management system in such human organizations as psychiatric hospitals. Social organizations behave like other organisms; they transform themselves through selective adaptation and new patterns—currently recessive—are emerging that promise basic changes.[3] Ellis Johnson caught the flavor of this phenomenon when he wrote: "In those large complex organizations the once reliable constants have now become galloping variables."[4] We are living in what Peter Drucker calls the "educated society" and this feature is the most distinctive characteristic of our time. Today the survival of the state mental hospital depends, more than ever before, on the proper exploitation of brain power. Warren Bennis envisions organizations as adaptive temporary systems of diverse specialists solving problems. He warned that "Bureaucracy, with its 'surplus repression' was a monumental discovery for harnessing muscle power via guilt and instinctual renunciation. In today's world, it is a prosthetic device, no longer useful. For we now require organic-adaptive systems as structure of freedom to permit the expression of play and imagination and to exploit the new pleasure of work" so necessary to meet the goals of a psychiatric hospital.[3]

THE CLINICAL EXECUTIVE

From the description of the functions of the modern state mental hospital and the organizational structure necessary to support these functions, it is evident that the superintendent must develop an equivalent leadership style. Because his management responsibilities, complex as they are, must be continually sensitive toward focusing all policy decisions toward the essential goal, which is the treatment and care of severely mentally ill patients, it is preferable that he be a well-trained clinician specifically experienced in the treatment of schizophrenia and chronic mental illness. Suffice it to say that I also feel it is a significant advantage in having an in-depth knowledge of personality development and a phenomenological awareness of the therapeutic process through having experienced individual psychotherapy. My reason for this preference is that despite all the pressures, conflicts, ambiguities, and decisions that the superintendent has engulfing him from the social, economic, and political environment, he must always be able to directly relate his emerging and changing policies as to their benefit for the individual patient. In administrating the tremendous amount of data upon which he must act, there is a constant tendency to lose sight of the patient and become entangled in the network of surrounding systems. With this as a backdrop, I will now focus on my conclusion that the superintendent, in order to administer the modern state mental hospital, must be technically competent in executive functions and have the personal characteristics of a facilitator. Fiedler's theory, and the research on which it is based, supports this conclusion.[5] He suggests that the leader's ability to use both instrumental and supportive leadership are a requisite for groups where tasks are in a state of change and also for groups whose members perform both structured and unstructured tasks. Instrumental leadership refers to a leader's ability to exhibit certain kinds of rational, intellectual behavior rather than social-emotional behavior. It describes an effective manager as one who plans, organizes, controls, and coordinates the activities of his subordinates. The supportive leader is a direct contrast to the autocratic leader. He endeavors to create a social climate in which each person will want to do his best and will not need compulsion. He provides general rather than close supervision and encourages his subordinates to use their own initiatives in handling the details of their job. It is also called "participative" leadership because such a leader participates with his subordinates concerning decisions that will affect them.[6] Etzioni, in his book *Complex Organizations,* has made the assumption that a shift from a custodial to a therapeutic hospital requires a change from a coercive to a normative organization, that is, from an autocratic to a democratic management structure.[7] Blau and Meyer emphasize that increasing reliance on specialized experts in organizations, which technological advances often make necessary and which rising level of education makes possible, constrains managers to abandon their prerogative of giving orders without explanation and to find other means of exercising leadership. In other words, where work is highly specialized, these attempts to assert hierarchical command authority often lead to conflicts between managers and their subordinates.[8] Every formal organization attempts to mobilize human and technical resources as means for achievement of its ends. However, the individuals within the system tend to resist being treated as means.[9]

The results of the failure of an adaptive change in leadership style as the organization moves from a closed to an open system is expressed explicitly by Lawrence and Lorsch: "Far too many administrators raised in one organizational setting and infused with the theory appropriate to it have wrought havoc by trying to apply it later in quite different settings."[10] Schulberg and Baker have raised two meaningful questions concerning the functions of the state mental hospital (which also imply different organizational structures): "Have these large institutions successfully adapted to the demands of the community mental health era, and consequently, are they ready to undertake new human service activities as well? Or do mental hospitals, still functioning as archaic facilities primarily oriented to inpatient custodial services of the past, finally need to be phased out?"[11] It is my assumption that one of the major factors continuing the archaic facilities, is not the lack of dynamically oriented integrative mental health services policy emanating from state departments of mental health, but their inability to effect change in the internal management system of the hospital in order to implement these policies.

SUMMARY

With the change in leadership of this particular state mental hospital, its management system went from one pole to the other, democratic to autocratic. Since professionals tend to move horizontally to other organizations if they are not satisfied in their work, the struggle in this particular case was short and quiet. I must end by stating that the process of bureaucratic formalization generated by succession in management is not inevitable; collective resistance can arrest it. Since this is a highly complex, sensitive, and difficult strategic procedure, it is rarely attempted.

REFERENCES

1. Paton, W. A.: *Accounting Theory.* Chicago: Accounting Studies Press, 1962.

2. McDonough, A. M., & Garrett L. J.: *Management Systems.* Homewood, Ill.: R. D. Irwin, Inc., 1965.

3. Bennis, W. G.: "Organizational Developments and the Fate of Bureaucracy" in *Readings in Organizational Behavior and Human Performances,* Scott, W. E. and Cummings, L. L., eds. Homewood, Ill.: R. D. Irwin, Inc., 1973.

4. Johnson, E. A.: Introduction to *Operations Research for Management,* McCloskey, J. F. et al., eds. Baltimore: Johns Hopkins Press, 1954.

5. Fiedler, F. E.: *A Theory of Leadership Effectiveness.* New York: McGraw-Hill, 1967.

6. Filley, A. C., & House, R. J.: *Managerial Process and Organizational Behavior.* Glenview, Ill.: Scott, Foresman, and Co., 1969.

7. Etzioni, A.: *Complex Organizations.* New York: The Free Press, 1961.

8. Blau, P. M., & Meyer, M. W. *Bureaucracy in Modern Society.* New York: Random House, 1971.

9. Burns, T., & Stalker, G. M. *The Management of Innovations.* London: Tavistock Publications, 1961.

10. Lawrence, P. R., & Lorsch, J. W.: *Organization and Environment.* Homewood, Ill.: R. D. Irwin, Inc., 1969.

11. Schulberg, H. C., & Baker F.: *The Mental Hospital and Human Services.* New York: Behavioral Publications, 1975.

Part III

THE POTENTIAL ROLE OF STATE HOSPITALS

Chapter 8

STATE HOSPITALS SHOULD BE REPLACED

J. Frank James, M.D.

WHY STATE HOSPITALS SHOULD BE REPLACED

Humanitarian Perspective

There was a time in this country in the 1950s and 1960s when moral indignation reached great heights. There were outcries for civil rights, against the war, against poverty, for humane treatment of the mentally ill. There was a President of the country who declared:

> I am proposing a new approach to mental illness and to mental retardation. When carried out, reliance on the cold mercy of custodial isolation will be supplanted by the open warmth of community concern and capability.[1]

There was a president of the American Psychiatric Association, Dr. Harry Solomon, who described mental hospitals as:

> antiquated, outmoded, and rapidly becoming obsolete. They are bankrupt beyond remedy. I believe, therefore, that our large

mental hospitals should be liquidated as rapidly as can be done
in an orderly and progressive fashion.[2]

Such humanitarian waxing following or parallel to war is
a historical pattern, occurring as if in reaction to the in-
humanity of war. The banner, however, can sometimes be carried far if there is a determination, a resoluteness of purpose,
and especially a large enough consensus. Our professionals have
lost the momentum. A transfiguration occurred, perhaps influenced by a hostile federal administration, by double-digit
inflation, by manpower problems, by the failure of community
programs to assume responsibility for difficult patients. These
have been large dragons to fight. Perhaps unconsciously, we
have fallen back to the security of our familiar bastions. With
much more caution do we rock the political boats by demanding—yes, "demanding" is a harsh word now—the best programs for our patients.

Others have picked up the banner. The legal profession is
in the forefront now. A *New York Times* article concluded with
this statement:

> The big state hospitals, even where they have not stunted their
> charges and demoralized their staffs, stand as monuments to our
> fears of those strange people inside. By hiding them away, at-
> tempting to break the connection between us, we deny their
> humanity and reject our own. The mental health lawyers are
> compelling us to find the means to bring as many of them as
> possible back among us. We have reason to be grateful, for our
> own sake.[3]

Groups whose motivations are not completely known,
such as the Church of Scientology and the Network Against
Psychiatric Assault, are placing us in a paradoxically defensive
posture. Ralph Nader demanded, "Planning should immediately be initiated for the long-range demise of state hospitals."[4]
A few patients themselves have succeeded in obtaining court
rulings to limit our use of state hospitals. A lament within the

profession is already being heard that the courts are interfering too much in our treatment practices. Unless we move positively in a humane direction, we are indeed vulnerable to court and legislated solutions that may not be best not only for us, but for our patients.

CLINICAL PERSPECTIVE

We should provide the direction, based first on our patient's needs, with clinical acumen that no other profession has. Let us examine their needs. It has been said that the system must be adequate to meet client's unmet needs, but not meet needs that the client can meet himself.[5] There is a large spectrum of patients with a variety of unmet needs, but for discussion, I will use three, large groupings.

First, and by far the largest, are people who need active treatment, frequently in crisis, sometimes requiring acute restrictive measures, and easily returnable to society. Some of these patients would have been sent to the state hospital in the past, but now community health clinics are treating them.

Second are the people who need more than crisis intervention or outpatient therapy, who tend to have unmet dependency needs, require lengthy treatment with or without psychotropic medication, and do not adapt well in society without help. Most of these patients would have been sent to the state hospital in the past and many would have stayed for lengthy periods. These are the patients that we have been criticized for in recent years, who don't need to be locked up, but do need more than they have been getting on the streets. Such efforts as the NIMH Community Support Program and other community programs, emphasizing case management, independent living, and rehabilitation, are specific for the majority of this group. On the more chronic end of this group are some patients who will still require lengthy stays in traditional community facilities, such as nursing homes or residential care.

Finally, a number of communities that are far enough along in their attempt to replace the state hospital system are reporting a small hard-core of patients that are not appropriate for most community-based programs. These patients are not just chronically disabled, they are also difficult management problems. We have found that their chronic psychotic illness is complicated by brain damage or characterological defenses, including acting out to the point of violence, manipulative behavior, and predilection to run away. This group has unmet needs to be controlled, and it needs to be treated aggressively. Kraft[6] described "a small, but persistent subgroup of patients," who were "chronic, severe schizophrenics" and estimated their number at one percent of the hospitalized patients. B. J. Smith[7] felt there was a two percent buildup in the hospital of "those whose emotional problems have left them with long-term diminished capacity for interpersonal relationships, vocational adjustment, educational pursuits, and social interaction." Marx[8] described three characteristics of his difficult to discharge patients:

1. A limited repertoire of instrument and problem-solving behaviors.
2. Powerful dependency needs.
3. A capacity to develop severe psychiatric symptomatology when confronted with mild to moderate degrees of stress.

W. G. Smith[9] found that neither state hospital or community mental health facilities were successful with "a small hard-core group." He stated that, "All the poor outcomes are concentrated in a few persons [which] suggests that a new attitude toward mental illness and a new emphasis in service delivery do not alter the basic process affecting the small hard-core of long-term patients." His small hard-core was only eight patients for a population of 700,000. If Manfred Bleuler[10] is correct that ten percent of schizophrenics should remain permanently hospitalized, we may be able, with further study, to estimate very closely how many of these hard-core patients we must plan for and provide leadership in taking care of.

Fresno County, California, with a population of almost 500,000 and a state hospital census as high as 600 at one time, has developed comprehensive, alternative programs. Nevertheless, for the past four years, there have at any one time been between five and eight extremely difficult-to-manage patients for whom we have still had to use the state hospital. There is constant pressure to admit more patients from the private sector and from clinic staff. Only strict criteria and a dedicated social service staff prevent the state hospital from being used inappropriately and much more frequently. So long as the state hospital exists, the pressure will be there to use it. Communities are reluctant to take on the responsibility for state hospital-type patients, but when the actual numbers of patients that are truly difficult to manage are identified, we may find that resources can be developed to take care of them.

ADMINISTRATIVE PERSPECTIVE

Those of us who are in clinical administration should also provide a better perspective on the organizational direction than any other profession, and also better than anyone who is only in administration or only in clinical work. Surely we have learned by now that individual community needs and individual patient needs cannot be appreciated by distant levels of government. Perhaps our greatest overall problem in mental health today is the inappropriate spread of responsibility for direct mental health services over three levels of government. Others[11,12] have pointed out this evolution of chaos, but a brief review may help to apply some practical recommendations.

State Bureaucracy

The first organizational error occurred when responsibility for the mentally ill moved from the local level to the state with the state hospital movement. The state-operated mental hospital may have been a necessary nineteenth-century movement. The state, at that time, was the smallest, viable funded unit of government that could assume the financial and organizational responsibility for humane care of the mentally ill. Then professionals concerned with mental illness were scarce, so that bringing them together in a centralized hospital was a progressive move. The population and population distribution of many states were such that centralized institutions were practical. State governments were small enough to allow for citizen involvement and closer supervision of institutions. In the nineteenth century, moral leadership was influential. The state hospital movement for asylum followed the Quaker penitentiary movement for penitence.

That age has past. Local governments and other local organizations have the capability of providing services closer to home and within a continuum of other resources. State governments have become ponderous, large bureaucracies that no longer have the capability of providing appropriate services and without any continuum of care. Professionals are now widely in the communities and not attracted to the state hospital-type of treatment. The population has grown so that many communities could justify a complete service spectrum. Most citizen involvement is now with local government, which is more responsive to local problems and more capable of providing supervision than distant state government. Today, moral leadership has given way to political realities, especially at the state level, which makes local government more sensitive to the problems created by the mentally ill.[13]

State government has demonstrated for 200 years that its priorities have not included the mentally ill; that it is not responsive to the needs of such an apolitical group, and that it is not receptive to the kind of clinical leadership, untethered by political ties, that is needed to accomplish the job. In reaction only to severe negligence and public outrage, have state governments made some improvements, but what of future whims of political and economic fates? The support of state hospitals will continue to fluctuate from state to state and from election year to election year. They will never fully obtain the support they need, never be completely accepted as therapeutic institutions, will never overcome the long-engrained stigma.

From the clinical administrator's viewpoint, we are aware of how easy it is to shift responsibility for a difficult patient to another level of government some distance away. We have all felt that feeling of relief, but we must also know how anti-therapeutic that rejection is. The term "state," all over the world, has come to mean a distant, impersonal power against which there is little hope to struggle. How difficult it must be for a patient to express gratitude or focus anger at the state. As our most vulnerable population to subjugation, the mentally ill find themselves in a web of nebulous bureaucracy not dissimilar from the fate of larger groups of people in other countries.

For those who would keep state hospitals open for the very difficult-to-manage, hard-core patients, we have shown, as clinicians and as administrators, that we do not draw the line very well. The courts are progressively taking that judgment away from us, but the time has come that we find the mechanisms to assure where the line is drawn. The number of patients that appear to need some type of longer-term, secure-treatment facility does not justify maintaining the split of a state-operated facility from the spectrum of growing community services, nor the discontinuity of those services that a patient suffers from being sent away.

Federal Naïveté

The second organizational error occurred in 1963, when the federal government, supposedly in reaction to the state's failure, implemented the federally-directed Community Mental Health Centers Act. For the federal government and our Chief Executive to declare a national policy against institutionalization was a great, historically significant move that, in fact, struck a great blow to the public's custodial orientation for the mentally ill. Even though relatively few of the proposed number of centers were established, the impact was of great value, as shown by reduction of state hospital use that followed, even in locations where there were no federal centers. This was an appropriate role for the federal government, which indeed should have the broad perspective of the needs of our society. That the centers should be directly operated by the federal government, however, has proved to be inappropriate. There were voices at the time who advocated for local control,[14] but the powers in NIMH were distrustful of local government and unfortunately had their way. The results were five mandated services totally unrelated to the goals of the act, to the problems of the institutionalized patients, the needs of the severely mentally ill, and the individualized needs of communities. That the five services mandated would take care of all the mentally ill demonstrated a naiveté seen only in those who are far distant from clinical realities. There were also voices at the time that advocated that aftercare be one of the mandated services,[15] but they also were ignored. This naiveté is not unlike the denial that clinicians frequently see in families that resist appropriate intervention. Man inherently resists acknowledging that mankind is less than divine. We have all seen this denial in the lay public for years, as represented by the reluctance of legislators to allocate adequate funding for the mentally ill, basically denying the extent and severity of mental illness. One of the great drawbacks to federal administration of mental health programs is, in fact, the dependence of support for federal programs on the Chief Executive. We have more recently witnessed the disastrous effect when the President is not supportive, if not outright hostile[16] to the needs of the mentally ill. This same denial may occur in some local governments some of the time, but not in all local governments at one time. There are enough concerned citizens and elected officals out there to insure that some will carry on the banner.

For three different levels of government to be responsible for direct services to the mentally ill is indeed an administrative nightmare in a local community. Decisions must often wait for distant supervisors. Duplication and triplication is common. A federally funded center may be in the same block as a community funded center, as is the case in Los Angeles. As a state hospital superintendent, I recall well the frustration of having patients return to the hospital after receiving no follow-up in the community, and I can understand well the state hospital staff who are now reluctant to give up the responsibility for their patients. On moving to the community in 1971, I recall one of the first negotiations I had to handle was among the clinic social worker, the state hospital social worker, the public guardian caseworker, and the state community services social worker— all of whom were responsible for the placement of the patient in question. We have since reduced this quadruplication to one case manager, but it was typical of the overlay of different levels of responsibility and the inefficiency of our disorganization.

The Community Support Program now being implemented by NIMH is as good a response as the federal government could be expected to pursue to the widespread criticism of the mental health center failure. It proposes better coordination and utilization of existing community resources for the support of dependent clients, an excellent goal for a particular group of patients. But it still will not serve the severely mentally ill, it will not answer all individual community needs, and it will have a difficult time merging with locally operated services. How many years will pass before enough clamor is made that someone up in the administration will realize that our first priority will have to be for the most severely disturbed. Meanwhile there will continue to be patients who will not take advantage of the Community Support Program, and if we rely on such a program, there will continue to be state hospitals. And meanwhile the integrity of the community mental health movement will continue to deteriorate, so long as our weakest link is not shored up.

The Community Mental Health Act of 1963 passed with

good intention, nevertheless did not address itself to the needs of the severely disabled. It did enable us to treat more people earlier. The parameters of government services for the mentally ill were widened. From the administrator's viewpoint, we know that with limited resources there must be a prioritization of services and a more efficient use of those limited resources. Federal or state government cannot perform this job.

Local Resistance

The failure of communities to provide alternatives to the state hospital has been well described. Part of this failure, as Lamb[17] has pointed out, was that they were actually mandated using federal funding for other purposes. Part of this failure has also been the inadequate funding of community programs that wanted to develop alternatives. In some areas where state hospital funding has been reduced, the funding did not follow the patients into the community. Part of this failure is also due to the stage of the process. Some communities are just now realizing that they must develop nontraditional services for their patients with recurrent illness; or for their patients who are excessively dependent, but resistive; or for their patients who are chronically difficult management cases. The technology is behind the movement.

Many of the failures in the literature inappropriately compare state hospitals with traditional community facilities. Allen[18] decried the fate of patients in board and care homes. Sylph and Kedward[19] found that the differences in terms of rehabilitation success between state hospitals and other facilities were negligible, but acknowledged that the other facilities "did not have a mandate to rehabilitate." Lawton, et al.,[20] found that a great many more patients could leave the hospital than there were appropriate facilities in the community to receive them.

Communities have not had the governmental mandate to develop alternatives, funding has been limited, and the technology for what kind of facilities has been slow to develop. Reimbursement by third party payers is still restricted to traditional nursing home facilities, including federal Medicaid. State licensing regulations have continued to provide only traditional categories of community facilities. Therefore, until state and federal barriers are overcome and appropriate facilities are available in the community, it is like comparing apples and oranges when such comparison is used to justify a "reorientation and revitalization of state mental health institutions."[21]

There are other resistances to community alternatives. There are still people who are fearful of the mentally ill and would always be content to have them locked away out of sight or at least zoned away. There are still economic concerns, such as the impact of facilities on property values. Local programs have a great deal of education and public relations to accomplish that they have not done. Local governments, depending on the orientation and experience of those in office at any particular time, may be very resistive to assuming a responsibility that the state has traditionally carried. Programs in some areas may, therefore, be slower to develop than in others. Peer pressure from other communities and from mental health leaders in other communities will eventually force progress. A peer Task Force of the Conference of Local Mental Health Directors in 1978 worked directly with the county mental health directors of the three most heavy state hospital users to develop plans to reduce state hospital use, advocated in the state legislature for special funding for those counties, and finally approached the governor to request that the administration release the funds available to the counties. The mental health directors in turn related this effort to their governing bodies, who approved the projects, which are now underway.

What may appear to be resistance to a distant government perspective may actually be related to timing and community priorities. Fresno County was one of 11 counties nationally chosen for a Community Support Program demonstration project, 100 percent federally funded, but funded for only one year. The local governing body, wary of one-time federal funding and more concerned with higher priorities, rejected the project. Three weeks later, the governing body appropriated a much larger amount of county funds to build a new facility that will, it is hoped, enable us to bring the few remaining state hospital patients back to the community.

Local government has a limited tax base, usually property taxes, to use for many local demands. This is a reality that cannot be overcome. Local funding alone cannot provide the resources that are needed to treat even the highest mental health priorities. Content to allow the state to assume the responsibility for the mentally ill many years ago, it is likely that the majority of local governments would do so again were there not some sharing of the funding responsibility. On the other hand, many communities have become sensitized to the needs of the mentally ill and, in fact, are putting in more than their share of mandated funds. In California, a recent poll of all counties showed that there is an approximate $9 million over-match, more county funds than are required by the Short-Doyle law. This is still not enough for the wholesale assumption of responsibility by local government. Elliot Sclar, a Brandeis University economist, has explained this circumstance, that the community:

> is a combination of institutions which relate to each other in a plane composed of a horizontal and vertical axis. Institutions relate vertically to other institutions with similar interests—institutions which are usually located somewhere else. These institutions usually also relate in a hierarchial way, with one controlling another. For example, the local church which relates to its national organization or the local mental health program which relates to the state mental health department are relating vertically. Churches relating to each other within a geographic area or local mental health programs which work with local clergy and schools are relating horizontally. The current breakdown in the community reflects the fact that vertical organization of social institutions is outstripping horizontal integration; as a result the feeling of loss of control which people voice so

frequently today is rooted in the fact that institutions which relate horizontally have little or no control over the necessary resources to affect local conditions. Now we plan to send patients for care into the same communities which lack much of the resources to support people both materially and spiritually.[22]

Sclar called for community programs to undertake "action and organizing that are today on the borderline of being considered unprofessional." To overcome local community resistance will indeed call for a new degree of activism on the part of local mental health professionals, if alternatives to the state hospital are going to be developed and if they are going to succeed.

Financial Perspective

In the face of inflation, a negative balance of trade, devaluation of the dollar, and a sluggish stock market, financial support for mental health appears to become a small consideration in the distribution of our national resources. Direct mental health costs have been estimated[23] to be one percent of the Gross National Product. Although small in comparison to other national products, the total cost of mental illness is still reported to be a staggering $37 billion, with current costs of care estimated at $14.5 billion. Surely that amount of funding can go far in solving many mental health problems, if the solutions are efficient and effective. Mental health leaders must actively pursue a course that will provide the best services as economically as possible.

Sheehan and Atkinson[24] reported that it was 16 percent less expensive to treat patients in a community center than in the state hospital. Gunderson and Mosher[25] pointed out that the highest cost of hospital-centered treatment was the loss of productivity that such treatment fostered, while "alternative facilities can promote much greater self-sufficiency and productivity among the inhabitants than would be possible in a hospital setting." Becker and Schulberg[26] pointed out that individual costs for hospitalization have risen because fewer patients have caused a concomitant rise in per diem expenditures. We have seen this in California where per diem rates have been set at $98 for 1979, as compared to $45 four years ago. Arnhoff, [27] in a poorly documented essay in *Science,* decried the cost benefit of community treatment. Kirk and Therrien[28] reasonably pointed out that, "No one knows the magnitude of the hidden community costs of community mental health or how they compare with the costs of hospitalization." These authors nor anyone else, however, have projected out the costs of hospitalization were we still using the hospitals at the same rate we were using them in 1955, when 77 percent of all patient care episodes were for inpatient care and there were over 500,000 patients in state hospitals.[29]

For the use of the same mental health dollar, we do know in Fresno County that the $2 million budget in 1969 paid for 73,000 patient days in the state hospital, while approximately the same budget in 1973 paid for 116,000 local community services. (See Table 1.)

Of great consideration is the prospect of the financial burden of National Health Insurance. Government may soon assume responsibility for the physical health of the citizens of this country. After original enthusiasm, there is now a more cautious note in the planning for such a national undertaking. Not enough attention has been paid to the mental health experience to learn from it. Government assumed responsibility for the mentally ill over 200 years ago and much can be learned from the unfortunate results of not providing the support that was needed to fulfill that responsibility. Prior to the implementation of universal health insurance, mental health leaders should demand that the commitment to the mentally ill be fulfilled first. At the same time, we can help show the way for a manageable health care system by developing a more cost effective mental health care organization than we now have.

The fee-for-service federal Medicaid model has poor cost containment ability, except to reduce the quality of service and

Table 1 The Turning Point—1973 Fresno County Mental Health

	1969–70	1970–71	1971–72	1972–73	1973–74	1974–75	1975–76
STATE HOSPITAL							
Days	73,451	48,742	25,377	1,845	419	2,029	2,329
Patients	350	200	100	10 aver.	3 aver.	6 aver.	6 aver.
Net Cost	1.314 mil	1.226 mil	$751,483	$30,750	$812	$79,673	$101,625
LOCAL SERVICES							
Direct	44,239	52,443	57,915	89,286	158,037	260,376	249,821
Indirect	1,299	1,402	6,132	19,866	36,454	54,254	83,894
Total	45,538	53,845	64,047	109,152	194,491	314,630	333,715
TOTAL SERVICES	118,989	102,587	89,424	110,997	194,910	316,659	336,044
TOTAL NET COST	2.402 mil	3.013 mil	2.682 mil	2.391 mil	2.825 mil	4.400 mil	5.279 mil

limit the number of practitioners who will participate. It does not encourage equitable distribution of services; the result is that practitioners are paid where they wish to practice, usually in large urban centers near university settings, rather than the money going where the greatest needs are. The budget is open-ended with no priorities and, therefore, no ceiling for control. We do not want to move in that direction. The current federal methods of allocating mental health funds is also difficult to manage. Pilot projects, declining grants, start-up funds, etc. do not represent a real commitment to the mentally ill. Local government, more and more, is resistive to those half-hearted offerings which essentially leaves local government holding the bag. Dissatisfaction with these mechanisms is apparently becoming widespread.[30] State government funding of state hospitals has been particularly whimsical, responding only when awareness of needs becomes widespread public knowledge or in reaction to media campaigns. I believe one of the reasons for this is that administrators in state-operated programs are in political double-binds that prevent them from advocating for patient care at the same level of government that also controls their personal fate and fortune. State level administrators, like state level patients, have virtually no constituency to support them as can be developed locally. State funding of community programs, more effective than federal, is also less related to community needs than to political circumstances and particularly to the power of individual legislators. The amounts of funding for any public endeavors will always, and perhaps appropriately, be regulated by the political process, but the mechanisms and accountabilities for each level of government can be made more responsive and efficient. Federal and state government are too far removed clinically from the realities that demand prioritization, too far removed organizationally to propitiously respond to community pressures, and too far removed politically to estimate the particular sequence and timing of each unique local program implementation.

What Should Replace State Hospitals

The "Small Portion" Left

State hospitals have been replaced to a great extent, according to statistics, which show a greater than 50 percent reduction and about a 10 percent rate of reduction since 1955.[31] In California, there is almost a 90 percent reduction of the mentally ill from 37,000 in 1955[32] to fewer than 4,000 now. This is a reality that state hospital proponents must face. With the decline, hospitals have become less cost-effective, and the milieu has changed, so that progressively the more difficult-to-manage patients remain. Therefore, we are not talking about replacing the state hospitals of 20 years ago when there were many patients who were easier to return than now. There are still some patients that can be returned with relative ease, if they are assisted to use existing community resources, since state hospitals have continued to be used inappropriately because they exist.

President Kennedy said, "If we apply our medical knowledge and social insights fully—all but a small portion of the mentally ill can eventually achieve a wholesome and constructive adjustment."[1] To replace the state hospitals, we must take care of that "small portion." This would appear to put the problem in much better perspective, since the numbers are really not overwhelming. We cannot move even this "small portion" from a bed in the hospital to a bed in the community without strong efforts to rehabilitate even the most difficult, or we will again start accumulating patients at one level. Historically this kind of build-up has been responsible for the failure of every effort, as resources at that level became overwhelmed. There must be movement. The Community Support Program, as proposed by NIMH, has worthwhile elements that will especially be helpful in assuring a better quality of life to patients who can now live in the community, but have limited resource-using ability. There is some danger in the "support" concept, which connotes a stable or static state that could foster dependency. If such be the case, as history has shown, there will be a gradual build-up of patients to such a level that they will eventually consume a disproportionate share of limited resources.

The Dynamic System

A more dynamic philosophy must be embraced in which movement is expected and is built into the system. Described previously[33] is a system in which three tracks should be visualized on which the patients are encouraged to progress to their optimal level of functioning. These are 1) a therapy-rehabilitation continuum; 2) a facility continuum; and 3) a social casework continuum. The following chart shows how these continua might theoretically function.

1. Therapy-Rehabilitation Continuum.   Both parts of this continuum are important components and could be independent to provide four tracks. However, because they must be closely operating together, I think it is helpful to see this as one track to emphasize that with this population they must be virtually inseparable. Also, it appears, with limited resources, most therapy resources are needed for the more acute patients. Perhaps when more resources are available to all of us, enough therapy can be devoted, with specialized techniques for chronic patients, to justify a fully complemented fourth track.

The "small portion" target population is almost entirely schizophrenic, with varying degrees of characterological defenses, and organicity. They do not generally relate well to traditional person-to-person or group therapy, although these approaches may be helpful to some as adjuncts. We must be careful not to generalize and try to see even this superficially homogenous group as made up of unique individuals. As Lamb[34] has pointed out, "It is important not to dismiss him as being incapable of psychotherapy." Lamb also mentioned some of the psychological concepts that are particularly helpful to keep in mind with chronic patients—regression, secondary

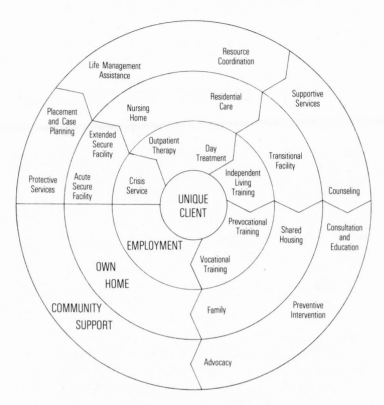

Figure 1   The Dynamic System (*Prepared by J Frank James, M.D., Joan Claassen, M.S.W., and Evert Christenson, M.S.W.*)

gain, and rationalization. A good background in psychoanalytic concepts will be continuously helpful for individual patients. All staff working with any mentally ill should have training in at least basic, analytic concepts. Since the unconscious of schizophrenic patients is qualitatively different from neurotics, all too commonly their bizarre, unconscious productions are ignored or actively suppressed. I have found that exposure of staff to Jungian ideas that allow for a broader universe of symbols to be helpful in stimulating communication with psychotic patients and providing them (the staff) with additional avenues for insight.

Medication, the most essential treatment at first, and probably the "great enabler" for all of community mental health, remains extremely important during rehabilitation. Without medication control, not of the person, but of the psychotic process, all other efforts will be futile. With most patients, as their particular medication need is titered and stabilized, medication should become peripheral to the continuum. It should not be the person-control that is used simply to keep patients in the community. With resolution or overcoming of internal conflicts and reconstitution of the ego, many patients will need progressively smaller amounts of medication. I follow some patients who remain psychosis-free on very small dosages of medication as their sleeping pill. Other patients, such as those on lithium, will require a definite blood level indefinitely. Other patients may progress to minor tranquilizers as needed to handle anxiety before it becomes overwhelming. The rehabilitation approach facilitates therapeutic interaction through transitional or intermediary objects. My impression is that a great deal of therapeutic activity occurs in the more casual, less threatening interchange between the rehabilitation worker–work tools and products–worker triad.

The main thrust, however, on the Therapy-Rehabilitation Continuum, is on progressively strengthening the ego and self-esteem through accomplishment. The higher the client can be taken on this climb, the less far he will fall when subjected to stress. There may be frequent hospitalizations during the first phase of rehabilitation, but as the client progresses, these will be fewer and regressions will be less severe. Within the system, rehabilitation is the crux, to prevent the build-up of chronic patients by moving them to higher levels of functioning. In our own program, the continuum consists of Independent Living Training, as the first level, followed by Prevocational Training, Vocational Rehabilitation, and Work Opportunity. Associated with these are socialization activities and continued therapy opportunities. These programs have been described in detail elsewhere[35] so only the philosophy is stressed here. Each community will have its own particular rehabilitation, especially work opportunity, resources. Replacement of the state hospital must include a dynamic progression of therapy-rehabilitation to avoid the dead-end and subsequent build-up of patients at one level in the community. Hogarty has stated it well:

> It is urgent that Federal and State Governments establish programs that provide a spectrum of supportive and restorative sociotherapeutic programs. Such services as would constitute the foremost priority for the chronically ill, particularly Schizophrenics, are currently the least endowed. They are often treated as stepchild services and are especially neglected in the comprehensive community mental health center.[36]

2. The Facility Continuum. This continuum is one that we have most avoided, either from denial of the needs in fear of duplicating the state hospital image or due to the delinquency of different levels of government to deliver the funding and regulations. The Presidential Commission's preliminary report proposed an Intermediate Care Facility for the Mentally Ill. A recent conference[37] of some of our best mental health professionals, chaired by John Talbott, M.D., was divided only on this item. Both viewpoints sounded a cautious note, "only in the context of a planned, integrated service system" and concern that it "might detract from the development of nonresidential rehabilitation and support services." The caution is understandable and we must indeed not exchange bed for bed only. However, we must face the reality of the need for facilities, not just one type, but a continuum with parallel tracks of rehabilitation and social services. Not facing the need, we are in another danger, as Maxwell Jones[38] questioned: "Can the development of hospital alternatives be left largely to chance as seems to be happening at present?" Leaving it to chance, an overloading and custodialization is already occurring. There are now more mental patients in Medicaid-supported nursing homes than there are in state hospitals.[39] Again we must avoid homogenizing the chronic patient, as we did with state hospitals, and appreciate the variety of living needs that the individuals have.

There should be room for innovation, with the spectrum running from "vacation resorts," suggested by Dickson[40] ("People who tend to run away could take ocean-liners.") to "non-therapy oriented custodial retreats."[41] A past president of the APA has reawakened interest in foster home programs.[42] A hospital-type facility "has a major role to play in the lives of all long-term patients whatever their placement,"[43] perhaps on a planned basis or at one stage in their progression. We need many varieties. The significant idea, like the other continua, is to not allow a dead-end to become overloaded. History has shown us this. From history we can also learn some lessons regarding who should operate the facilities.

In England, facilities, per se, began to be used in the early 17th century. Foucault[44] called this period "the great confinement." "Society's tolerance of madness had changed, with far-reaching effects, and the management of madness came to be bound increasingly to confinement." Parry-Jones[44] described the private madhouse system that ensued and flourished from the early 17th century to the last quarter of the 18th century. It was a business proposition, boarding unmanageable pauper lunatics at the parish expense in private dwellings. Not unlike our proprietary nursing homes of today, these dwellings became "truly notorious places," until the Lunatics Act of 1845 made it compulsory that counties build public-operated pauper asylums. The danger of the position in which we are even now finding ourselves by not addressing the issue is vividly quoted by Parry-Jones from a report by the commissioners in Lunay in 1844, after an inquiry into maltreatment at one of the private dwellings:

> The revocation or non-renewal of the license . . . would be most
> unwise and mischievous [because,] at this very moment every

> considerably lunatic asylum, both public and private, is full to
> overflowing; and if Hadock Lodge were to be at once shut up,
> a body of pauper lunatics not less than 340 in number ... all
> utterly unfit to be at large, would be instantly turned adrift and
> thrown back upon the already overcrowded workhouses or left
> in hopeless neglect and destitution to roam as outcasts through
> the community, to the terror and injury of the whole community.

The private system rapidly declined. Then, in the 19th century, the county asylums became overcrowded and fell into disrepute.

It is to be hoped that we can avoid the end results of that cycle by assigning the state its proper role of enforcing good regulations and the community developing a spectrum of facilities, and by actively participating in their programs. Even proprietary facilities must somehow be brought into the community network of services.

For the integrity of community mental health, let us focus on one level, the weakest link, our most-difficult-to-manage patients. After reviewing the variety of patients in state hospitals, Becker and Schulberg[26] concluded that "It is feasible to phase out state hospitals over a period of several years"; but they took note that only one group, the dangerous patients, would require, "a specialized facility ... to provide adequate security for the management of such patients." These are the hard-core patients that have been the main justification for keeping state hospitals open. There are not enough patients to justify the dual system.

It is imperative that within the spectrum of community facilities, a secure extended treatment unit be developed. The milieu of our acute inpatient units, which should be crisis-oriented, is already being destroyed by some of these patients who don't need to be sent completely away, but in the interim, revolve through the local acute hospital and make the rounds of all the other unprepared community facilities. It would be ideal not to need these, but idealistic to ignore the need. To keep state hospitals open for these patients keeps the door open for other patients who will continue to be excluded from the community inappropriately. Having these facilities in the community will avoid the greater stigma and rejection of state care. The benefits of the maintenance of contact with significant others and with community rehabilitation opportunities, and the closer proximity to the mainstream of society will offset the costs necessary to implement these facilities. As more and more criminal justice clients are diverted to mental health and since violence has become a more common expression of society's discontent, these facilities will, more and more, be needed.

These are the "small portion" that we are being held accountable for and that we can no longer ignore. The size of these facilities will be a critical factor. Maxwell Jones[38] felt that "a hospital population of fewer than 400 patients could develop a group identity to offset the familiar feeling of not belonging that is so characteristic of mental hospital patients." Parry-Jones[44] described the more therapeutic madhouses in the 19th century as "receiving up to 25 patients and this relative smallness, compared with the much larger county asylums, may have carried advantages." The original, namesake Dorothea Dix Hospital in North Carolina was a 20-bed infirmary. Studies previously mentioned indicate that the need may indeed be quite small. Further study should be made of the needs, and perhaps specialists in group relations should be utilized to help identify the optimal size, remembering as Gittelman[45] suggested, "Whenever possible, reduce the size of new facilities. In mental health, small is better than big. We must keep everything homey and human and avoid large institutions." It will be essential that prior concepts of cost-effectiveness oriented to custodial care must be replaced by cost-effectiveness related to rehabilitation. Let us raise our sights and demand the best level of treatment program for these, our most difficult charges.

3. Social Casework Continuum.   No array of services will succeed unless there are staff who care enough and are trained to reach out to the mental patient and are accountable for doing so. In one program, even when services were available, but no aggressive follow-up provided, 43 per cent of readmitted patients refused aftercare services and were lost.[46] The professions are being held accountable for those who are lost and we must identify individuals who are willing to accept that responsibility. These individuals require certain characteristics. Camus wrote about other-relatedness. Kolb[47] stated, "the most significant therapeutic arrangement that could be established is that of a pleasurable attachment to one or a number of staff members." In a very nice little article by Phyllis Santo,[48] called "Sacred Cows and Shibboleths," the attitude we seek is well-stated: "Casework can be fun, not only for the client, but also for the worker, when we enter into the relationship with our clients with zest, and with real understanding not only of their feelings, but of our own." There appears to be an increasing awareness of the need for and key function of the social caseworker or case manager. This professional may be called a variety of titles, the most recent one by Granet and Talbott[49] is the "continuity agent." They proposed that the person maintain a therapeutic position in the system, as well as being responsible for assuring that the patient bridges the gaps between various modalities of treatment. Our model in Fresno County is different. Established in 1972 by the transfer of state community social service staff to mental health, the program, called Advocare, has a primary mission of assisting and advocating for the patient across the gaps, without the role conflict of therapist versus caseworker. The staff have developed amazing skills at balancing the civil rights of patients, but somehow, still utilizing a variety of techniques to keep the patients in the system. We found the Title XX overall goals of "Self-Sufficiency and "Self-Reliance" as very helpful to the mission. In its first year of operation, the percentage of patients discharged from the state hospital who followed through on services in the community increased to 55 per cent under Advocare from 32 per cent under the state program. Since then the few state hospital patients remain on the service caseload and are regularly seen by their Advocare workers. Last year, the staff themselves initiated a "High-Risk Team," which carries a smaller caseload of the more difficult patients, and placed themselves on 24-hour call for these patients. For those who are considering a similar case management approach, you will find that priorities must be established for their valuable skills. The costs for all patients to have a separate case manager is prohibitive. An example of recent priorities for new clients (in addition to the high-risk patients and the chronically disabled) are: 1) History of recidivism to the local inpatient of more than two admissions in six months; 2) Diagnosis of schizophrenia, with history of not meeting medication clinic appointments; 3) Recent history of contact with the criminal justice system; 4) Skilled nursing facility placement, etc. With the clients, individual goals and objectives are initially identified and updated on a regular basis.

The case manager, by any name, is more than ever required as part of the replacement system for the state hospitals.[50] We can anticipate that communities will need this track, if they are to succeed and if they are going to be accountable for their patients.

The replacement of the state hospital should be a dynamic system of services, living arrangements, and monitor-advocates, which will allow patients to start from the lowest level of functioning, including the most difficult to manage, and move to their optimal level.

REFERENCES

1. Kennedy, J. F.: Message from the President of the United States relative to mental mental illness and mental retardation. Document No. 58, U.S. House of Representatives, 88th Congress First Session, Feb. 5, 1963.

2. Stratas, N.E., Bernhardt, D. B., & Elwell, R. N. : "The future of the state mental hospital." *Hospital Community Psychiatry,* 28:598–600, 1977.

3. Goodman, W.: "The Constitution vs. the snakepit." New York *Times* Magazine March 17, 1974.

4. Chu, F. D.: The Nader report: one author's perspective." *American Journal of Psychiatry* 131:775–779, 1974.

5. Test, M. A., & Stein, L. I.: "Special living arrangements: A model for decision-making." *Hospital Community Psychiatry,* 28:608–610, 1977.

6. Kraft, A. M., Binner, P. R., & Dickey, B. A.: "The community mental health program and the longer-stay patient." *Archives of General Psychiatry* 16:64–70, 1967.

7. Smith, B. J. "A hospital's support system for chronic patients living in the community." *Hospital Community Psychiatry* 25:508–509, 1974.

8. Marx A. J., Test, M. A., & Stein, L. I.: "Extra hospital management of severe mental illness." *Archives of General Psychiatry* 29:505–511, 1973.

9. Smith W. G., Kaplan J., & Siker D.: "Community mental health and the severely disturbed patient." *Archives of General Psychiatry* 30:693–696, 1974.

10. Bleuler, M.: 2nd Rochester International Conference on Schizophrenia reported in *Frontiers Psychiatry* 6:17, 1976.

11. Glenn, T. D.: "Exploring responsibility for chronic mental patients in the community." Conference on the Chronic Mental Patient, American Psychiatric Association, Washington, D.C., Jan. 11–14, 1978.

12. Christmas, J. J.: "Unresolved governance issues as barriers to care." Conference on barriers to mental health care, President's Commission on Mental Health, Airlie, Virginia, July 7–9, 1977.

13. Messner, E.: "Psychiatric observations of state and local politicians." *American Journal of Psychiatry* 134:1140–1142, 1977.

14. Musto, D. F.: "Whatever happened to community mental health?" *Psychiatric Annals* 7:510–522, 1977.

15. Yolles, S. F.: "Community psychiatry 1963–1974." *Journal of Operational Psychiatry VI:* 142–145, 1975.

16. Sabshin, M.: "Politics and the stalled revolution." *Psychiatric Annals* 7:98–102, 1977.

17. Lamb, H. R., & Zusman, J.: "In defense of community mental health." *American Journal of Psychiatry* 134:887–890, 1977.

18. Allen P.: "A consumer's view of California's mental health care system." *Psychiatric Quarterly* 48:1–13, 1974.

19. Sylph, J., & Kedward, H.: "Alternatives to the mental hospital." *Archives of General Psychiatry* 34:909–912, 1977.

20. Lawton, M. P., Lipton, M., Fulcomer, M., & Kleban, M.: "Planning for a mental health hospital phasedown." *American Journal of Psychiatry* 134:1386–1390, 1977.

21. Smith, D. C., Jones, T. A., & Coye, J. L.: "State mental health institutions in the next decade: Illusions and reality." *Hospital Community Psychiatry* 28:593–594, 1977.

22. Sclar, E.: "Girding for community care." *Behavior Today* 6:587–588, 1975.

23. Levine, D. S., & Willner, S. G.: "The cost of mental illness." Statistical Note 125, Rockville, Md.: Biometry Branch, National Institute of Mental Health, 1974.

24. Sheehan D., & Atkinson, J.: "Comparative costs of state hospital and community based inpatient care in Texas. Who benefits most." *Hospital Community Psychiatry* 25:242–244, 1974.

25. Gunderson, J. G., & Mosher, L. R.: "The cost of schizophrenia. *American Journal of Psychiatry 132:901–906, 1975.*

26. Becker, A., & Schulberg, H. C.: "Phasing out state hospitals—a psychiatric dilemma." *New England Journal of Medicine* 294:255–261, 1976.

27. Arnhoff, F.: "Social consequences of policy toward mental illness." *Science* 188:1277–1281, 1975.

28. Kirk, S. A. & Therrien, M. E.: "Community mental health myths and the fate of former hospitalized patients." *Psychiatry* 38:209–217, 1975.

29   Butler, H. J., & Windle, C.: *Evaluation overview - planning and deinstitutionalization.* Evaluation 4:38–41, Minneapolis: Program Evaluation Resource Center, 1977

30. Sharfstein, S. S., & Wolfe, J. C.: "The community mental health centers program: Expectations and realities." *Hospital Community Psychiatry* 29:46–49, 1978.

31. Bachrach, L. L.: *Deinstitutionalization: An analytical review and sociological perspective.* Washington, D.C.: Department of Health, Education, and Welfare. Publication No (ADM) 76–351, 1976.

32. Aviram, U., Segal, S.: "From hospital to community care: The changes in the mental health treatment system in California." *Community Mental Health Journal* 13:158–167, 1977.

33. James, J. F.: "Principles in developing a community support system." *Hospital Community Psychiatry* 29:34–35, 1978.

34. Lamb, H. R., et al.: *Community survival for long-term patients.* San Francisco: Jossey-Bass, Publishers, 1976.

35. James, J. F., & Claassen, J.: "A systems approach to the rehabilitation of the chronically mentally ill." 1st Annual Conference of the International Association of Psycho-social Rehabilitation Services, Philadelphia, November 1975.

36. Hogarty, G. E.: "The plight of schizophrenics in modern treatment programs." *Hospital Community Psychiatry* 22:197–203, 1971.

37. Talbott, J. A., Chairman: *Report and recommendations to the President's Commission on Mental Health.* The Conference on the Chronic Patient, American Psychiatric Association, Washington, D.C., Jan. 11–14, 1978.

38. Jones, M.: "Community care for chronic patients: The need for a reassessment." *Hospital Community Psychiatry* 26:94–98, 1975.

39. Report to the Congress by the Comptroller General: *Returning the mentally ill to the community, Government needs to do more.* Jan. 7, 1977, p.10.

40. Dickson, C. R.: "A modest proposal for a bold new approach." *Hospital Community Psychiatry* 29:41–42, 1978.

41. Rosenblatt, A.: "Providing custodial care for mental patients: an affirmative view." *Psychiatric Quarterly* 48:14–25, 1974.

42. Weinberg J.: "The chronic patient: The stranger in our midst." *Hospital Community Psychiatry* 29:25–28, 1978.

43. Steinhart, M. J.: "The selling of community mental health." *Psychiatric Guarterly* 47:325–340, 1973.

44. Parry-Jones, W. L.: "English private madhouses in the eighteenth and nineteenth centuries." *Proceedings of the Royal Society of Medicine* 66:659–664, 1973.

45. Gittelman, M.: "Coordinating mental health systems." *American Journal of Public Health,* National Association of Private Psychiatric Hospitals. 64:496–500, 1974.

46. Hall, J. C., & Bradley, A. K.: "Treating long-term mental patients." *Social Work* 20:383–386, 1975.

47. Kolb, L.: "Theory and clinical practice in long-term hospitalization." *NAPPH Journal* 8:27–32, 1977.

48. Santo, P.: "Sacred cows and shibboleths." *Social Work* 14:100–103, 1969.

49. Granet, R. B., & Talbott, J. A.: "The continuity agent: Creating a new role to bridge the gaps in the mental health system." *Hospital Community Psychiatry* 29:132–133, 1978.

50. Digman, P. R.: *The case for the state mental hospital.* Conference on the Closing of State Mental Hospitals. Scottsdale, Arizona, Feb. 14–15, 1974.

Chapter 9

STATE HOSPITALS SHOULD BE KEPT–FOR HOW LONG?

Henry Brill, M.D.

INTRODUCTION

It is now generally recognized that deinstitutionalization as applied to the state mental hospitals has fallen far short of expectations. What began as a manifestation of the highest moral, ethical, and legal motives has now been branded as a simple dumping of the mentally disabled from state facilities into the community and no more than a crude attempt to shift a financial burden from one agency of government to another. This has not led to an organized support for the mental hospitals as a better alternative, nor has it even halted the fall of their populations; according to provisional figures[1] the decrease was 11 percent in 1976. Yet questions have been raised about the theoretical and conceptual foundations of deinstitutionalization and about its practical aspects. The answers to these questions bear directly on the issue raised in the title of this chapter, namely, how long should the state hospitals be kept? Our conclusion will be simply that they should be kept till they have actually been replaced by alternatives that are equal or better.

In reaching such a conclusion we shall examine some of the theoretical background and assumptions underlying the movement and shall review briefly what actually happened in the course of implementation, noting especially certain barriers which were encountered. Our purpose in this will be to provide a foundation for our conclusions and to seek to benefit from the experiences of the past rather than merely to do a historical study, or even less to belittle the efforts that have been made. Finally we shall propose that the question be reformulated in more quantitative terms than has been the practice in the past and we shall give some examples of such data selected from the scanty information now available.

DEFINITION OF THE PROBLEM

Our discussion will deal largely with one function of the state hospital, namely the care and treatment of long-term cases because they account for the bulk of the population and the public image of these institutions is closely linked with the chronicity of their patients. Indeed the therapeutic effectiveness of the mental hospitals is called into question because of their presence. It may be noted however that these cases may be currently estimated at less than 155,000 and they are the residual of a flow-through of first admissions that have been coming at the rate of 100,000 to 150,000 per year. In other words, they are the unrecovered residual remaining from some 2,000,000 to 3,000,000 first admissions. Nevertheless, if these cases were removed the state facilities would become small, acute treatment centers, no different from all others. What we have to say about the state hospitals applies incidentally to other facilities of the same type such as county and veterans hospitals.

THEORETICAL AND OTHER BACKGROUND

Almost from their inception the state hospitals were a financial and political liability for state governments; it was with reluctance that the three branches of state governments passed the laws, decided the cases, and appropriated the funds providing for the frightening growth of these institutions. Given such a background, it is no surprise that there was universal support in 1963 when the federal government adopted the policy that the state hospitals should be replaced by community-based resources. No one could be opposed to such a policy on theoretical or practical grounds, and there was always the implication that federal dollars would follow federal policy.

The theoretical foundation for this policy, which was adopted in Great Britain as well as the United States, is drawn from a number of sources and unfortunately I know of no study that draws them into a pattern. I suppose such an account would in itself constitute a good-sized monograph, but for our purposes it may be sufficient to identify the following components:

1. A strongly environmentalist viewpoint that was well developed by the time of the French Revolution (St. Simon, Rousseau, etc.). This was further developed by such social scientists as Comte, LePlay, Mill, Durkheim, LeBon, and Tarde.
2. The development of a social psychology as exemplified by the Chicago School of the early 1900s. This group applied social sciences to psychological problems and are known through the work of such men as Ross and McDougall.
3. The application of social psychology and sociology to psychiatry, which created the new field of social psychiatry.
4. Wartime experiences (World War II) with early inter-

vention and recognition of environmental factors in the precipitation and control of mental symptoms.
5. Postwar concern with civil rights and liberties.
6. Federal initiatives in social welfare and social security.

Material drawn from such sources appears to have colored professional attitudes and provided the basis for the following specific assumptions with respect to the large mental institutions and their patients (a partial list):

1. That early treatment would now largely prevent chronicity.
2. That social recovery, at least, was possible in virtually all cases.
3. That the basic problems of patients were essentially social or psychosocial. In its most extreme form this view held that all involuntary and much voluntary hospitalization was unethical and immoral since there was no such thing as mental illness. This point of view had considerable influence on the courts and legislatures even if it was not fully accepted even by them.
4. That effective treatment was all but impossible in a large hospital.
5. That chronicity was the result of hospitalization and that community placement in itself would be therapeutic.
6. Once patients had been discharged into the community they would be able to rely on existing community resources and normal social assistance programs.
7. That the community would develop whatever additional resources might be needed once the patients were there.
8. The large infusions of federal funds for social welfare would end a major cause of hospitalization, namely poverty.

Space forbids our trying to deal with these point by point but as we follow the sequence of events we shall see how far these assumptions proved to be erroneous and how far they can be relied upon in future planning.

THE START OF DEINSTITUTIONALIZATION

For many years the major problem of the state mental hospitals was the endless increase of their population. The peak was reached in 1955 and with a figure of 559,000 for the United States and 93,600 for New York State, where the census had been doubling every 25 years.[2] Then, coincidental with the introduction of new chemotherapies, the increase was replaced by a slow decline nationwide and in other countries. In that year Congress created a Joint Commission on Mental Illness and Health and its report of 1961 strongly reinforced the current attitudes about the state mental hospitals. By that time the hospital population had been falling for five years at the rate of almost one per cent per year and had reached 535,000.[3] Nevertheless the commission did not come out for full deinstitutionalization. Instead they pointed out,[4] "Even with our best efforts to treat them in the early stages some schizophrenic, involutional, geriatric and senile patients will require continued care. These patients should be transferred [to] the proposed separate facilities for long-term patients."

They went on to propose that other chronic patients with physical disorders should be placed in the same facilities but the states showed no inclination to expand the spectrum of their direct services and within a few years took the opposite road toward deinstitutionalization.

DEINSTITUTIONALIZATION UNDER PRESSURE: THE 1960s

The enthusiasm for science and technology that characterized the 1950s had included the new psychotropic drugs but the

1960s were a period of social turmoil; the attitude toward technology had cooled and society looked for solutions to its problems in a rearrangement of its own structures. This rearrangement extended to the problems of mental disability. In some jurisdictions this took the form of outright administrative orders to place patients out of the hospitals. In others the pressures were more subtle, but the trend of case law, administrative policy and legislative action was unmistakable. The overall effect was a sharp acceleration of population fall. From less than one per cent per year before 1960 it rose to 7 per cent by 1969 and 13 per cent by 1974.[3] Even now the momentum seems to be retained and as late as 1976 preliminary data indicate a fall of over 11 per cent.[1,5] This is not surprising, since all the pressures continue in the same direction, namely to decrease admissions and increase discharges.

THE CURRENT PHASE: DEINSTITUTIONALIZATION IN THE 1970S

While the expectations and demands of the public continued unchanged into the 1970s the fiscal optimism of the 1960s was gone; inflation and unemployemnt were major concerns; cost containment was a watchword; and in many ways a narrower social point of view was manifest. Neighborhoods virtually sprang to the barricades at the prospect of any invasion by hostels or residential and treatment facilities for the mentally disabled. In my own county, a house was burned after it had been designated as a hostel for the retarded.[6] Demands for deinstitutionalization continue, but they are now coupled to preconditions. These are verbalized as preparation of the community for the patient, preparation of the patient for the community, creation of the necessary community resources, and planning to assure that the patient will adjust to the community. In practice this means that most people expect what amounts to a social recovery if the patient is to be placed, and they assume that if this does not occur someone is to blame. In this climate of public expectations there is likely to be a strong community reaction against individuals who stand out from the rest of the population because of oddities of appearance or conduct. In locations where feelings are aroused, the problem is magnified because alcoholics, confused older persons, and vagrants are all included in the rejected class. One has the impression that when turmoil breaks out on this issue it is originated and kept alive by a small group of citizens; but whatever the group dynamics, it has demonstrated the power to sweep the entire community with such force that few dare to dissent openly. The large literature on this topic has been well-reviewed elsewhere.[7,8] The public feeling that has been generated has been sufficient to bring about a major reorientation of planning in a number of states, including New York, where the administration has formally renounced "dumping" of patients.

SOME BARRIERS TO DEINSTITUTIONALIZATION AND OTHER IINTERPRETATIONS

With all of the forces aligned in favor of closing the mental hospitals and with no organized opposition, the question arises why, after almost 15 years, some 155,000 persons are still resident in these facilities. Why had the public seemingly ignored the process until the 1970s, when it had been more than half completed. It is fairly obvious that the barriers to deinstitutionalization were somehow intrinsic or inherent in the procedure itself, because even now the protests have to do with the practices and not the principles of community placement. With respect to public reaction, it would seem as if some threshold of tolerance had been exceeded and the public suddenly became sensitized even to long-standing situations that had previously aroused no opposition. At least this was the case with respect to a family care program that I had known for over 30 years and that had never created any problems. In the wake of the new attitudes about "former mental patients," this program suddenly came under attack without any provocation and was subjected to all of the community pressures that were now being applied to other types of placement. The long-stay patients had been expected to blend with the general population; this did not occur, and these former patients stood out even more prominently because many of them were forced by the pressures of social extrusion to gather in little ghettos, often in crime-ridden or otherwise run-down areas where they were an easy prey for the unscrupulous. They were not the beneficiaries of a normalizing contact with the community. I know of no attempt to track such populations, but from personal observation I find it unavoidable that these persons paid a price in health and lives for the poor living conditions, poor nutrition, and lack of protection to which they were subjected. The public was only too well aware of these alternatives to hospitalization and this led to another problem, that of families who put up with disruptive, irritable, actively hallucinated members to the detriment of children and family life in general—all this out of fear for the sick member.

A major barrier to the solution of the problems of deinstitutionalization is the legal independence of the former patients and of the persons who provide them services. In spite of their illness or incapacity, the patients are seen legally as fully capable even though this may be a polite fiction. Many of the cases simply disappear from sight, do not come to clinics or otherwise utilize available services. These patients take no medication and live literally in the shadows. The evils and weakness of this lack of control are illustrated by a case in our area when a newspaper launched a series of articles about a person who allegedly recruited such patients and in the guise of friendship took control of them and their funds, transported them about the state from one home to another, and even was said to have moved the body of one man from upstate to a local home after he had died. The conditions appear to have been very bad, yet it took some two years of litigation in addition to the activities of the press, to produce a conviction and a light sentence in this one case. This case aside, there are more than enough instances to show that for the mentally disabled in the community, money is not enough; it may only attract predators.

A related problem, which has had little discussion, has to do with the case of persons "similarly situated" in all respects except for the fact that they have not been identified by a stay in a mental hospital. How long could social and other governmental agencies continue to provide special care for ex-hospital patients and provide a different and inferior level of care for the far larger number of other mentally and emotionally disabled who may need the extra help just as much; for instance some 50 per cent or more of "skid row" populations fall into this class.

A major barrier to the process of deinstitutionalization may be labeled as fiscal disappointment. It has long been held that state hospital care is more costly than the alternatives, and I myself have been chided by political figures when I raised questions about that assumption. Yet experience does not seem to support the assumption that a decentralized service is less costly than a centralized one, other things being equal (types of patient and types of service). In New York State, for example, the mental hospital population fell by two thirds between 1955 and 1978, but the mental health budget for the institutionalized cases rose over fourfold and the total cost in public funds of community care can only be guessed at. Worse still is the fact that with all this increase in local and state expenditures, there has been no sign of fully meeting the needs. All types of service are considered to be underfunded and understaffed and there are even some areas of the state without locally based acute beds. Thus the lack of service for the former state hospital patient is only a part of a much larger problem and statistical data from across the country[5] and narrative accounts from Great Britain and elsewhere give ample evidence that the problem is general.

Another issue may be raised and that is the reality of deinstitutionalization itself. Some have alleged that what has happened, at least in part, has been a shift from one type of institution to another. Exact data will have to wait until large cohorts have been followed, but it is of interest that during a period when the U.S. state hospital population fell by some 200,000, the total institutionalized population of the United States remained quite stable (at a figure of about one per cent, that is 1,035 per 100,000 in 1950 and 1,046 per 100,000 in 1970).[3] It may be sheer coincidence, but it is interesting that the institutionalized population of Paris in the mid 1650s amounted also to about one per cent of the total population,[9] and a similar figure is reported for the institutionalized dependent Paris population in 1713.[10]

The curious stability of the American figures appears to be due to the transfer of cases among institutions. Thus the homes for aged and dependent persons increased their census from 296,783 in 1950 to 469,717 in 1960 and to 927,514 in 1970[3] at the very time that the population of the mental hospitals was decreasing by some 300,000. We shall make no attempt here to balance the figures but the literature on the subject is extensive enough to indicate that the transfer of persons from state facilities to other institutions is a very real one.[11,12,13] Much energy has been spent on recriminations and scapegoating in an effort to fix blame for these and other problems associated with deinstitutionalization. It is indeed tempting to become involved in the fascinating dialectic that has grown up around this subject, but another approach appears to be more useful.

SOME QUANTITATIVE ISSUES

It is probably wrong to ask merely whether we do or do not need state hospitals, because this allows for answers based more on principles, assumptions, or generalizations than on

observations and data. It may be better to proceed inductively
and to build up a definition as to what experience shows is
needed, how much is needed, and how much it will cost. Then
we can go on to ask how this may be achieved. At the start we
must note that the persons under discussion present a small
fraction of the total mental health problem and as such they are
easily lost to sight in the pressure of numbers in any overall
treatment system. They are the residual of some two to three
millions who came to the state hospitals as first admissions
during the past 20 years.[7] Their number shrinks still further in
comparison with the many million persons who may expect to
have some type of inpatient admission at some time in their
lives; not to speak of the four million who have some type of
patient care episode each year. Yet they have an importance far
out of proportion to their numbers, because of the cost of their
lifetime of care, their high visibility, and their human suffering,
which demands whatever relief is possible. They need a range
of services that the state hospital offers even when they leave
the hospital, and they represent a hard core of need for treatment places of some sort. For the most part their need is presented as part of the overall need for psychiatric treatment
places (or beds) regardless of the auspices under which they
may be operated or even their location. Unfortunately, the
literature on this topic is very limited and a recent survey found
only 29 English language references between 1964 and 1973.[12]
One of the most authoritative is that of Tooth and Brooke,
which actually dates from 1961. This projected a need of 180
beds per 100,000 of the general population (1.8 per 1,000). One
of the more recent studies concluded that for Great Britain
there had been nothing since that really replaced the 1961
report. In the United States, estimates of as few as 10 beds per
100,000 have been published, but I am inclined to believe that
the British figures are more realistic for the long run. These
range from 50 to 220 per 100,000. Some Scandinavian figures
range from 230 to 250 per 100,000.[14] As yet I know of no good
information on how these beds should be distributed among all

the various kinds of facilities nor on the actual volume of services that may be required to go with each type of facility. For example, the crucial issue of transportation is barely mentioned in discussions of a decentralized system.

The second question follows hard after the first one about total needs and total flow through of cases. That question is how many persons per 100,000 of the general population may be expected to become chronic under modern treatment conditions? (It is now generally accepted that some chronicity is unavoidable.) Here again the literature is scanty, but it seems that the figure of 6.8 per 100,000 per year is within the range of what one might expect,[15] although far higher and lower figures are quoted. Since these figures are cumulative for 10 to 20 years depending on life expectancies it seems certain that any system may expect the figure for long-term cases to build up to somewhere in the range of 125 per 100,000 in the course of years. The figures we have quoted here can be refined only as the result of experience and study; polemics are not likely to help.

CONCLUSION

It has already been demonstrated that it is possible by administrative action to abolish the system of state mental hospitals, but it has not been proved that this is the best alternative for all cases. In fact, considerable doubt is now being expressed on the subject. We now know that we were misled when we hoped that modern methods would reduce long-term disability to the vanishing point; what remains to be determined is what proportion of persons may have a better quality of life in a state hospital type accommodation and what proportion will do better in some type of community setting. It also remains to be determined what will be the real cost of adequate care in each of a variety of settings and what resources will be required.

While we are in the process of making these determinations, it seems well to remember that it will always be possible to decommission the existing hospital services and we have noted the powerful support this type of action has found. For the same reasons it will certainly be difficult or impossible to reestablish them once they are gone. Accordingly it would seem far preferable to retain them until they have been replaced by alternatives that are equal or superior to them rather than to continue to force their closure in the futile hope that a better system will arise spontaneously to take their place. We followed the British lead toward deinstitutionalization in 1963[16] and we might well follow their lead now. They have reduced their mental hospital beds by about one-third[17] as compared with our reduction of two-thirds in a shorter time, and they are now proceeding more cautiously with a continuous review of the results. I believe that we too should make haste more slowly and no longer use the criterion of sending people out or keeping them out of hospitals as the sole measure of success. We may be sure that as better alternatives are created there will be no problems about hospital closure—it will occur by default.

REFERENCES

1. Witkin, M. J.; Personal Communication. March 27, 1978 (Provisional estimates).

2. Brill, H., & Patton, R. E.: *The impact of modern chemotherapy on hospital organization, psychiatric care, and public health policies.* Proceedings of the Third World Congress of Psychiatrists. Vol III 443–37. Toronto: University of Toronto Press, 1964.

3. Kramer, M.: "NIMH psychiatric services and the changing institutional scene 1950–85." Washington, D.C.: Department of Health, Education, and Welfare. Pub. No. (Adm)77-443 Series B No 12, 1977.

4. Joint Commission on Mental Illness and Health. *Action for Mental Health.* New York: Basic Books, 1965.

5. Witkin, M. J.: "NIMH. state and county mental hospitals, United States, 1973–4." Washington, D.C.: Department of Health, Education, and Welfare Pub. No. (Adm) 76-301, 1975.

6. Carter, A. J.: "Site of hostel for retarded burns." *Newsday,* Jan. 16, 1978.

7. Bassuk, E., & Gerson, S.: "Deinstitutionalization and mental health services." *Scientific American* 46–53, February 1978.

8. Bachrach, L. L.: "NIMH deinstitutionalization: An analytical review and sociological perspective." Washington, D.C.: Department of Health, Education, and Welfare. Pub. No. (Adm)76-351, 1976.

9. Foucault, M.: *Madness and Civilization.* New York: Pantheon, 1965.

10. Ranum, 0. & Ranum, P.: *The Century of Louis XIV.* New York: Harper & Row, 1972.

11. Redick, R. W.: "NIMH: patterns in use of nursing homes by aged mentally ill." Statistical Note 107. Washington, D.C.: Department of Health, Education, and Welfare. Pub. No. (Adm)74-69, 1974.

12. Bachrach, L. L.: "NIMH: psychiatric bed needs: an analytical review." Washington, D.C.: Department of Health, Education, and Welfare. Pub. No. (Adm)75-205, 1975.

13. Schmidt, L. J., et al.: "The mentally ill in nursing homes. new back wards in the community." *Archives of General Psychiatry* 34:687–691, 1977.

14. Nielsen, J., & Nielsen, J. A.: "Eighteen Years of Community Psychiatric Service in the Island of Samso." *British Journal of Psychiatry* 131:41–48, 1977.

15. Fryers, T.: "New long-stay patients." *Psychiatry Quarterly* 8: No 4, 526–530, 1974.

16. Brill, H.: "The future of the mental hospital and its patients." *Psychiatric Annals* 5: No 9, September 1975.

17. Jolley, D. J., & Arie, T.: "Organization of psychogeriatric services." *British Journal of Psychiatry* 132:1–11, 1978.

Chapter 10

STATE HOSPITALS AS TERTIARY
CARE FACILITIES

James Barter, M.D.

The role of the state hospital has been fiercely debated in the past two decades with the shift in the locus of care of the mentally ill from institutions to community settings. It is suggested that state hospitals become tertiary care centers with responsibility for treating those whose care cannot easily be managed in the community. Characteristics of patients to be served as well as administrative and policy issues involved in such a transformation are discussed.

STATE HOSPITALS AS TERTIARY CARE CENTERS

There has been vigorous debate about the future role of the state hospital in the care of the mentally ill for the past two decades.[1,2,3,4,5,6,7] This is part of a broader social movement that has brought into question all forms of institutionalization for persons exhibiting socially deviant or unacceptable behavior and already has resulted in the establishment of alternative community programs for criminal offenders, alcoholics and mentally disturbed juveniles and older persons. The closing of many state hospitals was thus an inevitable part of this historical flow. However, in light of the recent furor raised concerning inadequate funding and lack of programs available for the deinstitutionalized mental patient, a reassessment is called for. We are now at the point where the role of relatively large state-funded facilities for the care of the mentally ill must be reevaluated. Are such institutions necessary? If they are, what should be their place in the existing and projected panoply of public and private services for the mentally ill?

The thesis of this chapter is that there is a continuing place for state hospitals and that they cannot exist in isolation from the rest of the mental health system of care. With planning and more broadly based political and financial support they can provide supplementary services that are a necessary component of and complement to good community based mental health programs. If the state hospital is to have a future, it must exist within a continuum of care for the mentally ill, and its role must be carefully defined, supported, and reinforced. Programs offered at the state hospital should compliment those offered at local levels rather than be in competition with them.

In this context it is proposed that state hospitals become tertiary care institutions providing specialized services for those patients whose needs are difficult to meet at the local level.

Tertiary care is defined as active treatment and rehabilitative techniques aimed at ameliorating the consequences of chronic mental illness. Integral to this concept is a research and training function that focuses on the management of chronicity and the rehabilitation of the chronically or recurrently mentally ill individual. Most importantly, a tertiary care facility must not be perceived as a dumping ground for those too difficult or too unsavory for community treatment. What is not being advocated is a purely custodial role for the state hospital in the care of the chronic patient.

WHO SHOULD BE ADMITTED TO STATE HOSPITALS?

There are three factors that influence admission to the state hospital: geography, target groups at risk, and systems analysis. Each differs in approach and orientation, but all have pertinence to the role of the state hospital as a tertiary care facility.

Geographical.   It is currently popular to designate specific geographical territories, e.g., catchment areas to be served by each state hospital. Often the hospital itself is further subdivided into geographical units serving a given section of a community, county, or state. A patient coming from a given location is admitted to the ward or program serving his geographical area. The geographical location of the hospital has a critical impact on the role it plays in relationship to local community programs. Obviously, a state hospital located within a major metropolitan area has the potential for being more integrated within a community mental health system than one remotely located. However, for administrative and political reasons this seems to be rarely achieved. Several specialized functions might be carried out within such an urban state hospital, which would complement or supplement the services offered by the community mental health centers in the area. These include a variety of inpatient services and aftercare, including medication follow-up, depending on the community needs. These, however, would not preclude the state hospital's becoming the major resource for tertiary care in the area served by the community mental health centers as well.

Rurally located state hospitals that primarily serve urban areas might find their role more restricted to the provision of tertiary care services than would those located in major metropolitan areas. Rurally located state hospitals serving rural community programs might offer a variety of services traditionally provided by community programs because of the problems of offering a broad range of specialized services in the rural community.

Target Groups.   A target group approach to defining the role of the state hospital concentrates on those individuals suffering from alcoholism, drug abuse, and chronic illness. It can also concentrate on those from specific age groups, such as children, adolescents, or the elderly. The major problem with this approach is that persons in each target group often need a full range of services, ranging from crises intervention through acute care to rehabilitation and aftercare services; these can best be offered within the context of the community program. In the model proposed here, only tertiary care services should be provided to these target groups by the state hospital.

Systems Approach.   In a systems approach, the needs of the clients being served are analyzed. Through orderly planning efforts, either existing services and programs are utilized, or new programs are developed to meet those needs. In either case, geographical and target group factors are considered in the planning. A systems approach does not make a value judgment about the relative merits of state hospital versus community based treatment, but rather looks at *all* the needs and *all* the resources and tries to determine where and how the particular needs of the patient at a given stage of his illness can best be met. Using this approach the role of the state hospital as a tertiary care institution within the context of a larger mental health delivery system can be clearly defined.

THE NEED FOR TERTIARY CARE

Given adequate resources, community mental health centers or local mental health programs can meet the needs of a large percentage of the mentally ill, including the chronically or recurrent mentally ill person. Criticism of the deinstitutionalization movement has been in terms of inadequate resources that lead to neglect of patients rather than pragmatic inadequacy. Neglect, when it occurs, has its roots in inadequate financing and planning of local programs, poor administration at all levels of government, lack of clear role definitions, poor coordination of services at the local level, and a variety of other assorted factors. That neglect is *not* the inevitable consequence of deinstitutionalization or of community efforts to treat the former state hospital patient in the community is demonstrated by the success of local programs around the country that have reduced state hospital populations by providing adequate services to the chronic mentally disabled population.

As an example, Sacramento County, California, (700,000 population) in 1969 sent almost a thousand of its citizens to state hospitals involuntarily. The inpatient population in state hospitals serving the county was approximately 750 persons. Through a deliberate policy of restricting admissions to the state hospital, accompanied by the development of alternative community programs, four years later the admission rate was less than 60 persons a year and the resident population had fallen to a low of eight persons. However, some individuals could not be managed in the community and there were clearly advantages to having the state hospital available as a backup for the community services. As a result, over the next four years, 1973-1977, the population of the state hospital increased and then stabilized at about 40 persons, with a rate of approximately 70 admissions a year. At the same time Sacramento County continued its innovative program for chronic mental patients.

There are then, clearly some patients or groups of patients for whom community programs are not feasible at a given point in their illness. These are, in a sense, community program failures. They include chronic deteriorated patients, actively aggressive and assaultive patients, and some individuals suffering from a combination of mental and physical illness so severe as to tax any of the local facilities. It is these individuals who vex most community programs, who consume enormous quantities of local treatment resources, and for whom the state hospital as a tertiary institution seems ideally suited.

CHARACTERISTICS OF PATIENTS NEEDING TERTIARY CARE

Chronic, Deteriorated Patients. This group of individuals offers a serious challenge to community programs. They require treatment programs provided by highly skilled and motivated staff of the type that have been developed in the better state hospitals. This patient population is not a homogeneous group and presents a panoply of medical and social problems. Symptoms exhibited by these individuals include mutism, catatonic excitement, enuresis, seizures, uncontrolled aggression, and rage. The severity and persistence of their symptoms taxes the resources of community programs, particularly if they are oriented toward rapid improvement and recovery of functioning. Treatment for this group takes a longer time than is offered by most community facilities and requires a variety of therapeutic approaches including medication, behavior modification, resocialization, and rehabilitation.

Aggressive/Assaultive Persons. A second group of individuals who frequently exhaust the resources of local mental health programs comprises aggressive and assaultive mentally ill persons. They are the people who make threats or assault relatives, friends, or other patients in community settings. Individuals with propensities towards specific sexual offenses are also included in this group of patients. One of their major requirements is for external control, which is difficult to provide in a community program since many of these individuals are referred after an assaultive act and enter treatment with a negative aura. If a community facility or program is not equipped to deal with such individuals, it is unfair (and perhaps unsafe) to expect it to accept the assaultive patient. A tertiary care facility, which has staff trained to manage such persons, may offer a much more effective treatment program.

The Physically Disabled. The third group comprises those persons suffering from significant and disabling physical or medical conditions. These persons require greater than usual nursing care and medical supervision. Examples include a psychotic, a diabetic double amputee, and a blind epileptic with paraplegia.

Some state hospitals have had excellent medical treatment available geared to this kind of mixed psychiatric/medical problem. Others could develop such an expertise if given a mandate and adequate support. Such care is not generally found in community mental health programs. In particular, so-called skilled nursing facilities are seldom equipped to deal with severe or mixed disablility and instead of help in coping with problems, patients are often provided care that barely enables then to maintain the status quo.

Theoretically, programs to meet the needs of the chronically disabled, the assaultive, and the physically handicapped mental patient could be developed at the community level. However, except in larger metropolitan areas, the number of such individuals in any one category at a given time is small enough to preclude their treatment on an economical or cost-effective basis. In these instances, centralization in a tertiary care institution makes ultimate sense.

There are other groups of patients who pose problems for local programs, depending on available resources. It is not proposed that the use of the state hospital as a tertiary care center be limited only to the groups mentioned. Instead, programs should be developed in as flexible a manner as possible so as to allow for the most appropriate "fit" with the local program.

It is well to remember that these groups of patients mentioned above cannot be treated as community castoffs. One of the dangers inherent in this proposal to convert state hospitals into tertiary care centers is that they might rapidly revert into abysmal custodial care institutions. Historically, this has happened when there has been inadequate funding, low staff/patient ratios, overcrowding, and inadequate facilities. If, in the process of transforming state hospitals into tertiary care centers, we do not remember these historical lessons, they may be repeated.

State hospitals functioning as tertiary care centers have a potential as research and training facilities. Factors leading to chronicity are poorly understood and new techniques for management and rehabilitation of the chronic mental patient are needed desperately. Incorporating a research and training component into a state hospital treatment program also could be extremely helpful in maintaining a sense of purpose and identity for the staff of the institution.

ADMINISTRATIVE ISSUES

In order to bring about the transformation of state hospitals into tertiary care centers there are a number of policy and administrative issues that need to be considered. Some of these have been mentioned or alluded to already, but others have not, and a separate discussion may be helpful at this point.

Single System of Care. One of the prime issues in mental health today is that of a commitment to a single system of care for the mentally ill. As it exists, there are multiple service systems at federal, state, and local levels dealing with the mental patient whose care is funded by public moneys. Rarely is the private sector considered or involved in the provision of public mental health services. Although the ideal of a single system has been espoused, it has not been fully realized anywhere. The dichotomy between the state hospital and the community treatment system or systems is an expression of this failure. Two systems have continued to exist for several reasons. Among these are special legislative interest, political pressure resulting from state employee organizations, and from local business leaders concerned about the economic impact of closure or reduction of the role of the state hospital. State hospitals often compete with local programs to provide the same services for the same patients. For instance, in some areas both state hospitals and local programs provide acute care and aftercare. It is inefficient and ineffective when two systems of care are maintained in such a competitive manner. It should be obvious that a better system would be one in which the role of the state hospital and the role of the community program were clearly defined as complementary and noncompetitive.

Administrative Role Definition.   Besides a commitment to a single system of care there must be a clearer definition of the respective administrative roles of each level of government involved in mental health care. A proposed model for such a definition would enable the federal government to be responsible for defining certain eligibilities and for assuring a certain level of funding through Medicaid or national health insurance. It would also oversee monitoring of quality control, cost effectiveness, and compliance with standards of care through regulation or other appropriate mechanisms. At the state level, the responsibility would entail statewide planning, priority setting, standard setting, and the provision of additional funding. The state also would have a role in monitoring local programs to assure programmatic quality, licensing of facilities and conducting evaluations of program effectiveness. The local level would provide the service delivery, with appropriate responsibility for a local plan consistent with the state plan, for administration and contracting for services, and for ensuring the quality of care. Protection of patients' rights and assuring adequate and humane treatment in accordance with federal and state guidelines would also be a local responsibility. Such a schema does not envision a direct treatment role for either the federal or state government. This raises the question of how to operate state hospitals, which have traditionally been a state responsibility.

One possibility is for state hospitals to be operated as though they were private corporations under state auspices. Each state hospital would have a governing board and an administrator responsible for its operation. Funding would derive from revenues collected for services provided under contract from local programs. All funding for mental health services would flow through the local program. The greater the number of units of service purchased by the local mental health program the larger the state hospital program. If one is to have a single system of care and define the role of the state hospital as one of specialized tertiary care, this sort of administrative arrangement is essential.

SUMMARY

There has been a great deal of change in the system of care for the mentally ill in the past two decades. It has evolved from a system based upon state-operated institutions to one of locally based multiphasic mental health services. In the process of change, the future of the state hospital has been fiercely debated, but in fact the philosophical trend has been towards an abandonment of that system of care for the mentally ill. In spite of this trend, the issues are not clear-cut. As the resources for community programs have fallen short of meeting the needs, and as the inadequacies of partially fulfilled promises have become more evident, there has been a reawakening of interest in improving the utilization of all available resources, including the state mental hospital.

No one advocates for a return to the traditional state hospital, or to custodial levels of care for the mentally ill. The future direction of the state hospital must be toward finding new roles and responsibilities complementary to community mental health programs. This contribution has explored one of these concepts, that of transforming the state hospital into a tertiary care center directed toward the care of those individuals who pose problems difficult to manage within community mental health programs. State hospitals can have a viable role in meeting this need.

REFERENCES

1. Bartz, W. R., Loy, D. L., & Cook, W. A. "Mental Hospitals and the Winds of Change." *Mental Hygiene* 55:266-269, 1971.

STATE HOSPITALS AS TERTIARY CARE FACILITIES   171

2. Lamb, R., Goertzl, V.: "The Demise of the State Hospital—A Premature Obituary?" *Archives of General Psychiatry* 26:489-495, 1972.

3. Schapire, H. M.: "The state hospital, what is its future?" *MH* 58:11–16, 1975.

4. Demone, H. W., & Schulberg, H. C.: "Has the state hospital a future as a human service resource?" in *The Future Role of the State Hospital*, Zusman, J., & Bertsch, E. F., Health, Lexington, Massachusetts: 1975.

5. Greenblatt, M., Glazer, E.: "The phasing out of mental hospitals in the United States." *American Journal Psychiatry* 132:1135-1140, 1975.

6. Steward, D. W.: "The future of the state mental hospital." *Perspectives in Psychiatric Care* 13:120-122, 1975.

7. Becker, A., Schulberg, H. C.: "Phasing out state hospitals-A psychiatric dilemma." *New England Journal of Medicine* 294:255-261, 1976.

Chapter 11

STATE HOSPITALS AS DOMICILIARY CARE FACILITIES

Richard N. Filer, Ph.D.
Jack Ewalt, M.D.

In considering what can be done with state mental hospitals, it would be very reassuring to know that the option to transform them into domiciliary care facilities was patient-oriented, with a determination to provide the most appropriate level of care to a significant number of patients in the psychiatric health care delivery system.

The steady decline in the number of patients in state mental hospitals since the mid-1950s has been attributed to various combinations of medical, social, economic, and political factors. Among the factors often cited are the advent of psychotropic drugs, admission and discharge procedures, alternative resources in the community, affiliation of community mental health centers with state mental hospitals, and increasing costs with resultant political pressures. Indeed, one of these, the availability of suitable alternatives in the community, has been touted in several studies to have significant potential for enabling the discharge of a majority of patients in state mental hospitals.

Alternatives to hospitalization fall into two categories: such noninstitutional programs as foster homes, and such institutional settings as nursing homes or domiciliary care facilities. In this regard, the 1966 study of state hospital patients in Texas found that 25 per cent were considered suitable for release from institutional care, almost one-third for transfer to some other form of institutional care, and the remaining 43 per cent were deemed suitable for further care in state mental hospitals.[1]

The finding in the Texas study that almost one-third of state hospital patients were considered suitable for transfer to another form of institutional care is consistent with the assessments of other health care delivery systems. The Veterans Administration experience is a case in point.

A gradual, but steady decline in the number of beds designated as psychiatric in the VA hospital system has occurred since the late 1950s. This culminated in a reduction of psychiatric beds from 54,345 in 1967 to 28,173 in 1977. During this period the annual number of admissions increased from 71,076 to 161,969. This change has been associated with an increased attendance at mental hygiene clinics, day treatment centers, and day hospital programs. The total number of these visits increased from 753,553 to 1,613,974 annually. The number of psychiatric hospitals has decreased from 41 to 23, as these institutions have broadened services and been converted to a general medical and surgical mission. The psychiatric services in GM&S hospitals had only 12 per cent of the psychiatric beds in 1967; they now have 60 per cent.

But during this transition era another interesting phenomenon emerged that has implications for the concept of transfer of patients from one institutional setting to another. There was increased utilization of domiciliaries for outplacement of patients from psychiatric hospitals.

Domiciliaries represent the original programs in the Veterans Administration and derive from 1866 legislation establishing Soldiers' Homes for disabled veterans. Originally the domiciliaries were converted barracks and there was little intent to provide medical care. During World War I some medical facilities were created, and these became more developed when the Veterans Bureau became the Veterans Administration in 1930. Additional legislation in 1946 increased the emphasis on medical services with the establishment of the Department of Medicine and Surgery, but the domiciliaries continued essentially as a protected residential program. Interestingly, as the transition phase of the VA psychiatric hospital described previously was taking place, the VA domiciliary program also experienced significant statistical changes. The peak patient membership was in 1956 when the average daily census was approximately 17,000. Since that time, the number of patient-members has been progressively decreasing, and in 1976 the census was slightly over 9,000. The loss has not been to state veterans homes since total state domiciliary census has also fallen from 8,228 in 1966 to 5,562 in 1976.

While there was a steady decline in the overall population in designated VA domiciliaries, the proportion of patient-members with a diagnosis of psychoses has increased by almost two-thirds between 1969 and 1975, a significant trend in the type of patient being served by the VA domiciliaries. Moreover, the proportion whose principal diagnosis is psychiatric, in general, has increased from 36.3 per cent in 1969 to 50.9 per cent in 1975. This trend primarily reflects the increasing percentage of patient-members previously cited whose principal diagnosis is psychosis, ostensibly in partial or full remission. The average length of stay was 2.86 years in 1967, compared with 3.61 years in 1975, increasing gradually in that interval. This consistent trend may reflect the concurrent increase in the proportions of psychiatric patients for the same time period.[2] Apparently, then, there has been an increasing tendency for the Veterans Administration to view a different kind of institutionalization (domiciliary) as more suitable for many patients than continued stay in psychiatric hospitals. In spite of these statistics, a recent study of the VA health care system by the National Academy of Science reported in 1977 that several thousand patients located in VA psychiatric hospitals would benefit more from a domiciliary setting.[3]

The truth is that for many years large psychiatric hospitals (both state and VA) have incorporated and provided a domiciliary function. This was provided under a variety of names, i.e., continuous treatment wards, custodial care, milieu therapy, etc.; but essentially it was a label for a program or nonprogram prescribed for all patients residing in psychiatric hospitals who were not designated as "acute care" patients. It was inevitable that the mere fact that a network of domiciliaries existed within the VA health care system would invite consideration for their outplacement potential as pressures increased in the VA psychiatric hospitals to find suitable outlets for an essentially residential type of population that did not need hospitalization or nuring home care, and yet did not quite, for one reason or another, meet the necessary criteria for adjustment within other community alternatives, e.g., return to family, independent community living status, or personal home care (foster home) placement.

The VA Domiciliary Program is designed to provide necessary medical treatment and comprehensive professional care for eligible, ambulatory veterans in a residential type setting. The program is directed toward those veterans who are disabled by age, disease, or injury, and are in need of care but require neither hospitalization nor the skilled nursing services of a nursing home. To be entitled to domiciliary care, the veteran's disability must be chronic in nature, and he must also be incapacitated from earning a living and have no adequate means of support.

The primary focus of the domiciliary had traditionally been to provide food, lodging, and limited medical care in an institutionalized setting. The time period between 1967 and 1975 represented a change in the emphasis from custodial care to a therapeutic community concept stressing more preventative health services, rehabilitation, and restoration.

According to the most recent statement of the mission of

the VA domiciliaries,[4] both medical and professional care programs are tri-level in order to meet the needs of all patient-members. Veterans requiring prolonged care in a protective environment benefit from preventive medicine and rehabilitative measures. For intermittent residents, special behavioral and medical rehabilitation is provided on a temporary basis. Short term restorative services enable other residents to return to community living within one year.

Although utilization of the domiciliary as a more suitable institutional placement for large numbers of patients "living" in VA psychiatric hospitals did increase over the past decade, it apparently did not completely solve the problem since the National Academy of Science study reported in 1977 that thousands of patients suitable for domiciliary placement still remained in VA psychiatric hospitals. Why?

An analysis of the VA domiciliary system in the early 1970s indicated that there were several dimensions that should be considered in assessing the appropriateness of an institutional setting for outplacement of hospital patients. These include: availability of these facilities, absolute size of the facility, age and type of architectural design, geographic location, and mission and program that could be provided in that institutional setting.

In considering the future role of domiciliary facilities in the VA health care system, several of these factors are being assessed, and these may have implications for development of domiciliary facilities in a state hospital system.

The absolute size of an institution may reinforce many of the negative attributes of institutionalization, depersonalization, apathy, and increased dependency, among others. When a large institution is also physically separted from other components of the health care system, additional negative influences develop. There is, for example, a tendency to develop a self-contained community. It is easier and more economical to bring all services and resources to the institution rather than have institutional members go to normal sources in the outside community. Recreation is brought to the institution, libraries, chapels, and stores are brought to the institution, and work opportunities are created within the institution, often artificially. People come to visit friends or relatives at the institution, if they come at all. Specialized health care resources are developed within the institution rather than the residents going to the array of health care resources utilized by the outside community. The list goes on, but the effect is a self-contained community to which the resident becomes adjusted, while this institutional experience promotes a diminishing capacity to cope with the realities of the outside world.

To the factors of size and geographic isolation of institutional facilities, add the ingredient of increased proportions of aging patients in the health care system along with chronicity and long-term care. Can effective, high quality long-term care be consistently rendered apart from acute care? Should long-term care be in isolation from acute care?

An alternative model proposed, and now partly implemented by the Veterans Administration consists of providing long-term care in a setting adjacent to and integrated with acute care facilities. This assures an ease of transfer between levels of care for both acute and long-term care patients. The availability of high quality acute care in the same institutional setting engenders excellence in long-term care as well, and the recruiting of competent personnel is significantly easier. High quality professionals are not usually attracted by the prospect of treating and caring solely for long-term patients in isolation from acute care patients and facilities.

The scope of problems and services required by isolated long-term care facilities alone is insufficient to provide the academic and research environment necessary for health manpower training. In association with acute care programs, however, long-term care adds technical breadth and depth of understanding.

There are not, in fact, two groups of patients—acute and long-term—but rather patients whose needs cover a continuous spectrum from the most acute to the most long-term. Patients move back and forth along this spectrum, especially because the so-called long-term patient has a very high incidence of acute disease episodes. Only by an integration of acute and long-term facilities can the acute care needs of the long-term patient be adequately met.

But, in what kind of physical facility can this integrated program take place?

The suitability of existing structures for utilization as domiciliary facilities raises another question that can be frankly stated: Should a population be fitted into inappropriate buildings because the buildings are there, or should facilities be remodeled or built to meet the needs of the projected resident population? The answer, of course, is that existing facilities have to be appraised in terms of meeting life safety codes, patient privacy standards, and other factors related to program requirements. The wide variety of existing facilities will require some hard decisions in this regard.

The Veterans Administration, in response to this question, has recently embarked on a new approach. Having ascertained that it would be extremely costly to remodel most existing domiciliary facilities to attain adequate fire, safety, and privacy standards, a new type structure has been designed. This facility will be limited to 200 beds at any one location. Barracks or ward-type facilities will be eliminated in lieu of one-bed or two-bed rooms. Four 50-bed pods will be connected by a central support area. Each 50-bed pod will also contain one multiliving unit (a living room, bedroom, kitchen combination) and each 50-bed pod or the total facility will be constructed to be completely convertible to a nursing home care unit if necessary in the future. For example, a kitchenette in a residential 50-bed pod could become the nursing station, storage rooms then become staff offices, etc. The facility will, then, rather than being designed as a fixed residential facility become a flexible, extended care facility where the needs of a population with changing requirements can be adequately met. Medical care will be on an ambulatory or outpatient basis. To the extent possible, recreation and social activities will be community oriented. These small, flexible facilities will be geographically dispersed and become an integral resource within a medical district for appropriate planning purposes. Ground has been broken for the first of these flexible extended care facilities at the Wood VA Center, Milwaukee, Wisconsin. Several others are scheduled to follow.

In summary, it appears that a substantial demand for provision of an appropriate residential care function will continue in the psychiatric health care delivery system for the immediate future. Utilization of existing state mental hospital facilities for this purpose should consider factors that are related to negative aspects of institutionalization, i.e., size, geographic location, and architectural design. However, if institutions are necessary during our time, could not the positive aspects be emphasized?

The desire for security sometimes becomes so intense that it obscures deeper and more significant values—individuality and personal dignity. In a sincere effort to aid people in need, societies for years have established various forms of institutions, and sometimes the desire to provide security has become the ultimate goal. One of these kinds of institutions is the sheltered environment or congregate living situation. It would be foolish to say that such institutions should not provide, insofar as they are able, a measure of security. This can be done in part by assuring shelter, food, medical care, and a variety of comforts; but it would be equally inappropriate to stop there. Such things may keep people alive, but not necessarily living. A basic component of a congregate domiciliary facility is, then, a program designed to add meaning and direction to the residents' every day living in order that each individual might maintain respect of self, purpose of being, and personal dignity.

Food, clothing, shelter, and medical care can be given to people directly in large or small measure, but not personal dignity—it is not man's to give. This must come from within the individual. Similarily, we cannot give another self-respect.

What we can do, however, is to establish the conditions that encourage and make it possible for a person to maintain or regain his own feeling of respect for self and personal dignity.

REFERENCES

1. Pollack, E. S., & Taube, C. A.: "Trends and projections in state hospital use." Chapter 2 of: *The Future Role of the State Hospital.* Zusman, J., & Bertsch, E. F., Lexington, Mass.: Lexington Books, 1975.

2. *Social, demographic, and medical characteristics of patient-members in VA domiciliaries: 1976–1975 Profile.* Controller Patient Census Monograph No. 3. Washington, D.C.: Veterans Administration, August 1976.

3. National Academy of Sciences, NRC, Study of Health Care of American Veterans. Committee on Veterans Affairs, U.S. Senate, Committee Print No. 4, June 7, 1977.

4. Department of Medicine and Surgery Manual, M-2, Part XIX, Washington, D.C.: Veterans Administration, May 15, 1970.

Chapter 12

STATE HOSPITALS AS COMMUNITY MENTAL HEALTH CENTERS

Francis A. J. Tyce, M.D.

The socially dysfunctioning individual is one markedly out of phase with the society in which he lives. His dysfunction can be protean: mental illness, neurosis, marital or family problems, problems in functioning in living as a child, adolescent, adult, or aged person. His dysfunction can be caused by vocational problems, illegal behavior, rebelliousness against the system in which he lives. It can be caused by abuse of chemicals or alcohol, or by developmental disabilities, learning disorders, helplessness in the problem of adjusting to the life experience, loneliness, rejection, alienation by others of different racial and ethnic origin. This list is far from complete.

If a state hospital is to attempt to deal with some of these problems, what qualities should it possess, or try to develop, to assist those people I have called socially dysfunctioning?

The state hospital

1. Should be *visible* to the community it serves. They should know where it is.

2. Should be *accessible*. It should be easy of access and on a good transportation pattern.

3. Must be *available,* 24 hours a day, 7 days a week. A good hotel can be very visible, a skyscraper, in the middle of the traffic pattern. But if it is closed, it is useless, it is not available. It is a hollow promise.

4. It must be *penetrable*. It should be devoid of restrictive policies and easily penetrated by consumers, relatives, visitors, media, other community facilities. All subunits within the hospital should be easily penetrable also.

5. It must be *credible*. Those who work in the hospital and those who use it, should believe in it.

6. The hospital must be *cooperative*. It should find it easier to say yes than no in its relationship with the community and the community facilities it works with.

7. The hospital must be *sensitive*. It should be attuned to all small cries from the community.

8. It must be *responsive*. That is, it must be willing to act.

9. It must be *flexible*. It should be willing to adapt.

10. It must be *changeable*. That is, it must be willing to give up old ideas.

11. It must be *creative*. That is, it should be willing to be imaginative.

12. It must be *courageous*. It must be willing to accept challenge and not regard timidity as a safer and desirable goal.

13. It must be *accountable*. It must be responsible to its consumers, its staff, its community, and its central authority.

If the hospital has the physical qualities of visibility, accessibility, availability, penetrability, and has developed credibility, and if it continually strives to be cooperative, sensitive to the community needs for the treatment of its socially dysfunctioning, and most importantly responsive to these needs, and is willing to be flexible, changeable, then creative and courageous in trying to meet these needs, what programs might it develop for the socially dysfunctioning person?

For the mentally and emotionally ill, a psychiatric service should contain the following elements:

I.

    a. An inpatient adult psychiatric service in mixed male, female open units that are regionalized—that is, each unit individually serves a certain fixed geographic area in the hospital's total receiving area. These geographic subareas should contain a community mental health center. Traffic between the inpatient unit and the area and community agencies it serves should be open, encouraged, reciprocal, and continuous.

    b. A *day hospital* for patients who need not stay in hospital at night.

    c. A *day nursery* attached to the day hospital. Since most patients in a day hospital program are women and married, they need somewhere to leave their preschool children while they use the day hospital. The day nursery is available to patients who use other services on the hospital campus, to staff people who have a family crisis, and to volunteers who work regularly at the hospital and cannot find or afford regular babysitting.

    d. *A night hospital.* Unlike the day hospital, which will be a separate entity, each psychiatric unit can function as its own night hospital.

    e. *Adolescent inpatient services* with an accredited school program supervised and staffed by the local school district.

    f. *Outpatient services.* Again each psychiatric unit

should provide outpatient services to those who need it after previous hospitalization. Thus continuity of care is provided by the team that looked after the patient in hospital.

II. For the socially dysfunctioning who are chemically dependent, the following programs are needed:

   a. *A detoxification service for those chemically intoxicated.*

   b. *A chemically dependency unit* closely associated with the detoxification unit so passage from it to the treatment unit is easy and expected.

   c. *Night programs* for the still-working alcoholic.

   d. *Diversionary programs* designed in conjunction with local judges so treatment rather than punishment is an alternative which can be chosen by the chemically dependent lawbreaker.

   e. *Half-way houses* for those who can now work in the community but still need supervised living arrangements.

   f. *Programs for the families of the chemically dependent* so they can develop understanding and support in his efforts to obtain sobriety.

III. *Residential care* for the developmentally disabled—both long-term programs designed in conjunction with the local school district, and respite care for shorter periods of time. Here the resident lives at home and can be admitted for short periods when the parents need assistance in learning to program for him at home, or when there is parental illness, a family crisis, or simply a need for a parental vacation.

IV. *A geriatric service* for the dysfunctioning aged person, living alone, with family, or in a nursing home. Admission should be made easy, and close cooperation and swift assistance given. This will persuade both nursing homes and family to take the patient back when they have the assurance of good followup care.

V. *Residential care for the criminal offender*—another group of socially dysfunctioning people both young and adult. The state hospital has had long experience in helping to create and design new programs. It is sensitive also to the effects of total institutionalization, and has a lot to offer in helping to set up programs in community corrections.

VI. *Special programs.* The state hospital might help to set up programs for statewide needs, for children services, forensic services, and special diagnostic and treatment services.

VII. *Vocational and rehabilitation services.* Years ago in Phase I in the history of state hospitals, the hospital may have provided good medical care and benign custody.

With the advent of new drugs and new techniques, the hospital moved to Phase 2 or the removal of symptoms and revolving admissions. Now in Phase 3 we know good medical care, the removal of symptoms, is not enough without vocational counseling, habilitation, and rehabilitation that makes certain the patient on discharge is vocationally independent and self-supporting.

Thus the state hospital may respond to local, regional and statewide needs and create a diversity of programs. But to do this it needs money and personnel. I doubt any state hospital has ever had, or will have, enough money. The hospital should, therefore, have a basic unchanging commitment that it will strive to give away all, or as much as it can, of its operation back to community control, community funding, and community programming. If completely successful the "hospital" image disappears, the diversity of programs remain, and the campus becomes a regional resource for the socially dysfunctioning person.

Personnel in state hospital systems is equally as scarce as money, but here we can substitute ingenuity, and historically state hospitals have demonstrated ingenuity. If personnel time in patient contact can be increased, then their usefulness expands. The commitment should be that all clinically trained personnel, psychiatrists, psychologists, social workers, nurses, rehabilitation workers etc. should remain in positions of direct patient care. If the director of the hospital is a psychiatrist, he should have clinical responsibility for one psychiatric unit. To maintain highly trained professionals in administrative work only is to waste their expertise and leads to program design without continuing experience, and communication by memoranda—a time-consuming, self-deceiving, relatively inaccurate method of communication.

Responsibility and authority to act and to participate in treatment planning should be forced down and down, through staff levels down to and including the patient and his family.

Why should the psychiatrist spend time compiling the psychiatric history? This should be done by the patient's primary nurse with the patient writing his own developmental history and autobiography, which is then included as part of the psychiatric history. Who knows his developmental history better than the patient? The psychiatrist can read it later. The patient's autobiography should include his list of the problems that have brought him into the hospital and his ideas for their solution. To make the best use of time, remember that confrontation with the patient and his problems should be direct and speedy. Transference develops rapidly when time is short.

All interviewing with patient, patient and relatives, and patient and community resources should be interviewing shared with the patient's primary nurse and other team members who will work with the patient. Single interviewing between patient and psychiatrist means that information gained has to be passed on often incompletely to other staff after the interview, and time is thus wasted.

I have yet to meet a patient who will not discuss his problems frankly with a number of people in the room, when he realizes all are interested in helping him. This does not obviate single staff to patient psychotherapeutic treatment sessions when it is indicated.

Discharge summaries can be written by the head nurse or unit director, read, and countersigned by the unit psychiatrist, freeing more of his time for patient contact and teaching on his own unit.

The work of recreational therapists can be greatly expanded by inviting young people or resident volunteers to live in the units with patients, in exchange for room and board. They can devise one-to-one or group activities for patients during the empty times when staffing is lowest—the evenings and weekends.

VIII   *Hospital Interface with the Community:*
       The hospital should be seen as an important ally in the communities' attempts at social engineering and social planning. Sound trusting relationships must be built between hospital, law enforcement, courts, media, and citizen groups, all of whom are prime movers in community action and can support or deter new programs for the socially dysfunctioning person.

What happens to a state hospital if it becomes a center for mental health?

It is predictable that
1.   Hospital census will go down. See Table 1
2.   Admissions will go up. See Table 2
3.   The percentage of voluntary admissions where people seek treatment volitionally will go up. See Table 3
4.   Outpatient visits will increase. See Table 4

To have said at the beginning of this chapter that I was describing a particular hospital would have been presumptuous, to have described as existing, what actually does not exist would have been delusionary.

I'm sure I have described nothing that is not familiar to

Table 1 Rochester State Hospital Ending Census
1960–1977

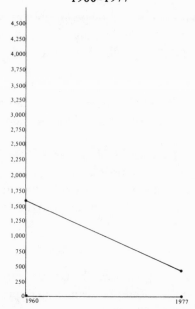

Table 2 Rochester State Hospital Total Admissions
1960–1977

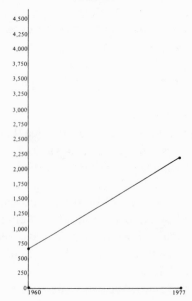

Table 3 Rochester State Hospital Informal Admissions
1960–1977

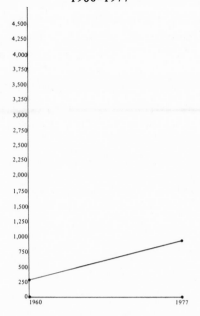

Table 4 Rochester State Hospital Out-Patients
1960–1977

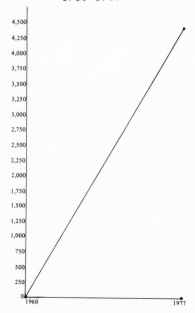

you who work in state hospitals across the country, but if some aspects are unfamiliar, the operating policies and the program activities described all exist on the campus of the state hospital where I work which I hope make it with other cooperative but autonomous programs based on the campus a center for mental health and a least restrictive alternative in the treatment of the socially dysfunctioning individual in southeastern Minnesota.

Part IV

THE FUTURE OF STATE PSYCHIATRIC SERVICES

Chapter 13

STATE HOSPITALS — SOME VIABLE OPTIONS

Robert deVito, M.D.

At this time in the evolution of the community mental health movement, state mental health authorities throughout the country are being confronted with the awesome task of having to decide whether to continue or to close state mental hospitals and developmental centers. During the last five years, the State of Illinois Department of Mental Health and Developmental Disabilities (IDMHDD) has exercised both options by closing one of its larger state mental hospitals while continuing several others. In FY 78, however, the department reduced its total hospital count from 28 facilities and 3 annexes (facilities under the same administrative control of but physically distant from the parent facility) to 28 facilities and 1 annex by utilizing some newer concepts in facility transformation; i.e., (1) annex closure with transfer of function to both the public and private sectors and (2) annex conversion to a whole new set of functions with transfer of original functions totally within the public sector. In the first instance, the department closed a small residential triage and treatment center (Malcolm X Mental Health Center) for acutely mentally ill citizens from the South Side of Chicago in October 1977 by transferring those functions to a private sector facility (Chicago Osteopathic Hospital) and to the center's parent facility (Tinley Park Mental Health Center). Staff from the Malcolm X Center were given the option of returning to the Tinley Park facility so as to maintain a smooth transition in mental health services without a negative economic impact to individuals or to the involved community. In the second case, the department converted a 700-bed residential habilitation facility (Lincoln Annex) for the severely and profoundly developmentally disabled (DD) to a 750-bed medium security prison (Logan Correctional Center) in December 1977. In this conversion 10 different IDMHDD facilities participated in the transfer of DD residents while 3 different department facilities and the newly created correctional center took part in the transfer of staff. As in the case of the Malcolm X closure, staff were given the option of remaining within IDMHDD or transferring to the Department of Corrections. Most elected to stay in the Lincoln area, either at the parent facility (Lincoln Developmental Center) or at the Logan Correctional Center, thus minimizing the potential negative economic impact on the town of Lincoln.

With the success of these two ventures, the department has embarked upon a new conversion plan, involving the transformation of two facilities, to be completed by June 30, 1981, subject to legislative approval. This chapter will focus on the historical background, systems planning, strategizing, and anticipated implementation scheduling of this project as a means of illustrating some of the major theoretical and pragmatic considerations that should be borne in mind in catalyzing moves of this dimension.

During my first year as director of IDMHDD, it became evident that while administrative and programmatic reasons should form the basis of any plan for facility change, economic and political factors become the dominant forces that determine whether or not a plan will "take." A flat organizational model that stresses the importance of input and feedback from both within and outside the organization, stimulates creativity and innovation and provides the primordial seedbed for major change. Adopting a basic administrative philosophy such as a general systems approach allows the mental health authority to organize and integrate this input into a cogent, cohesive plan for presentation to the executive, legislative, and judicial arms of government as well as to a broad spectrum of professionals, interest groups, media, and involved lay public. Given six fundamental options from which to choose (viz.: continuation without change; continuation with alteration; partial closure; complete closure; partial conversion; and total conversion), the mental health authority has a number of fascinating variations on these six themes to consider. The Tinley Park-Illinois Institute for Developmental Disabilities (IIDD) double conversion plan reflects some of these variations.

HISTORICAL BACKGROUND

As one of a number of states on the vanguard of the community mental health movement of the 1960s, Illinois has gradually evolved from an institution-based system of care to a geographically distributed system of services for the mentally disabled and substance abuse populations. With 24.3 per cent of its proposed FY 79 budget of $427.2 million appropriated directly to the community in the form of grant-in-aid and purchase care moneys, one cannot depict the Illinois system as being community-based at this time, even though it is clearly moving in that direction. The double conversion plan is an attempt to catalyze this movement, while simultaneously mounting solutions to some vexing long-term problems, best outlined as follows:

1. Lack of state-operated residential programs for the mentally ill (MI) *in the inner city,* particularly in view of the

fact that three of the nine highest poverty areas in Illinois are in the South Side of Chicago (Subregion 11) and represent a major referral source for inpatient MI services at the Tinley Park Mental Health Center, located in a southern suburb of Chicago with inadequate public transportation from the city. Hence, individuals from the South Side of Chicago have to be served outside their community, which fosters isolation from family and community, impedes linkages with community agencies, and makes it difficult for subregion staff to coordinate residential and outpatient follow-up services.

2.   Lack of residential services for the DD population in Region 2 (a nine-county area that includes metropolitan Chicago, its suburbs, and exurbs). Currently there are 1,926 state-operated DD beds in Region 2 while 2,050 or 53 per cent of Region 2's DD residents are being served in state-operated facilities outside Region 2.

3.   Lack of programmatically sound, adequately staffed services for the multiply-handicapped DD population at the Dixon Developmental Center (DDC), a large, isolated IDMHDD facility in a small rural town in Region 1A. Currently, of Dixon's total residential population of 1,506, 1,214 have families living in Region 2. Some of their physical settings are bleak, unstimulating, and expensive to renovate. In addition, local administration has experienced a continuing difficulty in recruiting and retaining qualified professionals, particularly medical and nursing personnel.

4.   Underutilization of the IIDD building in Chicago's West Side Medical Center. IIDD is one of IDMHDD's two nonresidential facilities, devoted at this time to DD training and research, as well as to diagnostic assessment of prospective Region 2 DD residents. The department currently funds the more than 70 full-time IIDD staff, some of whom also have teaching and research appointments at the nearby University of Illinois Circle Campus, with whom the department developed a formalized working agreement in September 1977 aimed at

fostering research and training in the area of DD, identifying the Institute for the Study of Developmental Disabilities (ISDD) as the jointly supported nidus of this effort.

5.   Lack of Joint Commission of Accreditation of Hospitals (JCAH) accreditation at Dixon as well as inability of many of Dixon's programs to meet HEW Title 19 certification standards at this time. With the lowest staff-patient ratio in the department (1.18 to 1), Dixon is the farthest away from both accreditation and certification.

SYSTEMS PLANNING

Given the five long-term problems described above, and in view of executive and legislative support for the changes at the Malcolm X and Lincoln Annex Centers, the department began searching for some far-reaching solutions to these problems in the spring of 1977. This entire process was given further impetus by the Tinley Park mayor, the village trustees, and the chief of police, all of whom had pointed out to the department leadership that village residents were extremely fearful of the dangerous psychotic patient population that had been treated at the Tinley facility since 1968. While the department had partially resolved this issue by strengthening the mental health programming on individual treatment units at Tinley as well as by increasing the size of their security force, the village representatives continued to press for an intrinsically less dangerous treatment population at the facility. As a consequence of a careful analysis of these problems, the department designed a plan outlining three principle initiatives. The plan was submitted to the governor on February 7, 1978, and formally approved by him in a major speech at the annual meeting of the Mental Health Association of Greater Chicago on March 13, 1978. The chief elements of the plan are as follows:

A.   *The Conversion of the Tinley Park Mental Health Center (TPMHC)*

   1.   Transfer of the inner city (Subregions 11 and 12) adult MI programs from Tinley Park MHC to the IIDD building.

   2.   Transfer of the subregion (Subregion 14) adult MI program, a 45-bed unit, from TPMHC to the Manteno MHC, a DMHDD facility located in the southern part of Subregion 14.

   3.   Transfer of the 40-bed children and adolescent (C+A) program from TPMHC to the Chicago-Read and Madden Mental Health Centers or to other state-operated C+A programs within Region 2.

   4.   Negotiation with the Departments of Corrections, (DOC) and Children and Family Services (DCFS) to relocate the Tri-Agency (DMHDD, DOC, DCFS) Adolescent Treatment Program from the Tinley Park Campus to a site elsewhere in Region 2.

   5.   Development of 500 beds for the severely and profoundly developmentally disabled on the Tinley Park Campus, 420 to be run by private sector DD agencies, the remaining 80 to be run by DMHDD; specifically, the Howe Developmental Center, a modern, fully accredited 400-bed facility, located immediately west of the Tinley Park Mental Health Center. The plan calls for the Howe Center to extend its administrative domain to include the additional 80-bed unit and to serve as an alternative service provider should private sector agencies be unable or unwilling to run a 420-bed residential DD program.

   6.   Deeding or leasing some of TPMHC's buildings or land to the village of Tinley Park so that the municipality could opt either to provide services for 420

DD residents directly or to contract with private sector DD agencies to do the job, with DMHDD acting as a catalyst in the process.

B.   *The Conversion of the Illinois Institute for Developmental Disabilities (IIDD)*

1.   Relocation of IIDD's research, training, evaluation, diagnostic, and early intervention programs from the IIDD building to another location within the West Side Medical Center of Chicago (within one to six blocks of the present site).

2.   Relocation of three tenant (non-DMHDD) programs currently housed within the IIDD building to sites agreed upon by the tenants and DMHDD.

3.   Continued DMHDD funding for the more than 70 IIDD staff as part of the department's commitment to support a strong research and training effort in collaboration with the University of Illinois Circle Campus, identifying the Institute for the Study of Developmental Disabilities as the focal point of this effort.

C.   *The Systematic Improvement of DD Programming at the Dixon Developmental Center (DDC)*

1.   Phased transfer of 390 DD residents from the Dixon Center to the publicly and privately run DD programs on the Tinley Campus.

2.   Phased transfer of 176 additional DD residents from Dixon to other publicly operated DD facilities, primarily in Region 2, making a total of 566 transfers, so as to reduce Dixon's census to a total of 940 residents.

3.   Decelerated reduction of Dixon staff during the resident transfer process to a target of 1,457 full-time equivalent positions, eventuating in a 1.55 to 1.00 staff-patient ratio (a substantial improvement over the current 1.18 to 1.00 ratio).

4. Coincident capital improvements, aimed at transforming large, open-bay, barracks-like physical environments to home-like, modular settings.

5. Development of active, ongoing training and education programs for all staff at Dixon, which together with the staffing and capital improvements, will lead to the kind of facility-wide programming that should result in JCAH Accreditation and Title 19 certification for all habilitation units.

IMPLEMENTATION STRATEGY

Experience with the Malcolm X and Lincoln Annex Center changes demonstrated that timing, flexibility, and public discussion with full media coverage are three essential elements in successfully implementing any plans of major significance. From a timing perspective, it is useful to first share a prospective conversion plan in writing with the governor and his human service agency liaison staff in order to assess its administrative, programmatic, and political viability and to determine, from a media standpoint, whether it should be viewed as the governor's plan or the department's plan with the governor's support. From a practical point of view, a governor's plan usually receives top executive priority whereas a departmental plan may or may not. In the case of the Tinley-IIDD double conversion, the governor announced it publicly as his plan and, hence, it has had the swift and full support of the Bureau of the Budget (BOB) and the Capital Development Board (CDB), two key branches of the executive arm of state government. Following the announcement of the plan on March 13, 1978, I appointed the department's associate director for DD services as head of a task team to catalyze the implementation of this plan. Conceptualizing the task team as a temporary organizational unit with program, management, and budgetary expertise, one can now visualize that the department has a focal group in place, which can serve as a clearing house for the enormous amount of data that is being generated with reference to the plan.

A pivotal part of the timing of the process is communicating the plan's principle elements to individuals and groups who are likely to mount significant opposition to it, such as employee unions and community interest groups. In the Tinley Park-IIDD project, I met with the union leadership prior to the governor's making a final decision, supporting their request to transmit their input to the governor directly. By so doing, they were given an opportunity to reshape the plan and even scuttle it early in the process. In like fashion, the governor had an opportunity to evaluate the merits of their opposition as well as my analysis of counterarguments to the plan. Their principle reservations centered around concern about employees' rights, job loss through layoffs, and loss of union membership. Their fears were somewhat lessened by management commitments to honor all existing labor-management contracts and to make every attempt to avert layoffs by the use of attrition, particularly at the Dixon Developmental Center. As a follow-up to my conferences with the union leadership, the task team project director named a representative of the American Federation of State, County, and Municipal Employees (AFSCME) to be an ongoing member of his 11-man implementation team. The result of these moves, up to this point, has been a close working relationship with all employee unions, despite ongoing differences of opinion as to the specifics of the plan.

Given strong executive support for this project, the task team has scheduled public hearings in the Tinley Park, Near West Side Chicago, and Dixon areas as well as legislative, interest groups, and media briefings relative to the plan. At the writing of this paper, the department has held three public hearings, and several briefings with some fascinating results. While there has been surprising public, professional, media, and political support for this plan, there have been small but highly vocal pockets of criticism, primarily from unions, some DMHDD employees, and special interest groups. The greatest opposition thus far, has emerged from the Near West Side of Chicago, in a meeting called by local citizens, dissident DMHDD employees, and union representatives, all of whom objected to the transfer of psychotic acting-out patients from Tinley Park to the IIDD building with its alleged security problems and relative lack of recreation space. Administration officials, including task team members, responded by noting that because IIDD is located in a high crime area of Chicago, the department, in collaboration with the Chicago police department, has elevated the authority and responsibility of DMHDD security officers in that area to that of Chicago police officers. Beyond this, the fact that IIDD is located in a major medical center suggests that professional recruitment, particularly medical and nursing, should be more successful than is currently the case at the Tinley Park Mental Health Center; hence, better programming, more effective individual treatment interventions, and it is to be hoped, fewer unauthorized absences. In all public meetings, the department has stressed the flexibility of the plan, inviting interested parties to recommend alternatives to change those aspects of the project with which they are in disagreement. What is emerging as a consequence of these strategies, is a steadily mounting crescendo of support for the plan, despite its controversial nature. There is no doubt however, that continued public hearings, particularly in the Near West Side will be necessary, if the plan is to come to fruition.

Chapter 14

STATE PROGRAMS–ADVERSITY, OPPORTUNITY, AND SURVIVAL

Lee B. Macht, M.D.

"I curse you; may you live in an important age." wrote Nikos Kazantzakis[1] making reference to an ancient chinese statement. This applies to our era in the mental health field as well. For this has been a time of transition between the period of the large custodial state hospitals and the attempt to develop community-based programs while we upgrade smaller hospital inpatient units. We[2] believe it is a watershed period in a historical sense; one where we stand to lose a great deal or may make a quantum leap in the humane, progressive care of the mentally ill. As with any such historical period of transition we can expect both adversity and opportunity to emerge. This chapter will highlight both elements and will examine the historical parallels to the decline of moral treatment and what needs to be done to ensure that community mental health, and with it modern psychiatry, especially in public practice, survives. It will take the position that our greatest enemy is despair and hopelessness and that psychiatry must reemerge as a profession with leadership in the mental health field, taking an advocacy role, along with others, in the interest of highest quality patient care both in community and institutional programs. With this we must become politically active to achieve these goals, while we develop a new cadre of clinician administrators[3,4] to fill leadership positions. We will briefly examine the Massachusetts experience over the last several years as a case in point as we further develop these ideas.

CASE ILLUSTRATION

The Commonwealth of Massachusetts has a long history of providing services to the mentally ill. Hospitals in this state were at the forefront of the moral treatment movement. Like most states, we developed large custodial institutions after the decline of moral treatment. However, we did develop a psychopathic or receiving hospital early in this century and began some community clinics even before 1955. In that year our state hospital census was 23,000 and ever since it has steadily declined to our present 4,900. In 1966 the state enacted legislation providing the framework, but not the dollars, for a system of community-based care in 40 catchment areas of the state. Over the years some 13 federal community mental health center staffing grants were obtained. The budget grew slowly and most of the resources were allocated to the institutions and not to community programs. In 1970 the state hospitals were geographically unitized but it was several years before linkages began to develop with the catchment area programs and only presently that the areas are beginning to take responsibility for their state hospital units. The range of community mental health services is spotty across the state. Some areas are very advanced and many offer only minimal services. For years the legislature debated whether to have community programs or institutions and saw it as an either-or situation. For years resources were moved from the institutions to the community to the point where staffing in the institutions became difficult.

There was only a minimal appropriation for community services.

In 1975 we arrived in Massachusetts at a major crisis point. The state was on the brink of financial disaster, the new governor had promised no new taxes in his campaign, the tax base had eroded, Medicaid and welfare costs had soared. In addition there was a new chairman of Ways and Means in the state House of Representatives, a new Secretary of Human Services, and a new interim Mental Health Commissioner (LBM). Fortunately the Undersecretary of Human Services, a psychiatrist (Donald J. Scherl) had remained in office and proved to be a major support to the whole agency. The Department of Mental Health was beset by the usual problems of civil service, hiring, freezes, year-to-year funding, hospital certification, judicial consent decrees, problems with contracting for services, etc.; in addition, the governor and legislature called for a 20 per cent reduction in funding for all agencies, including mental health. Staff began to leave programs and could not be replaced because of freezes and problems with recruitment and morale reached an all-time low.

Under the leadership of the commissioner, a psychiatrist, a number of steps were taken. Working with the Secretary and Undersecretary of Human Services he was able to convince the Secretary of Administration and Finance and the governor and legislature to allow for hiring of clinical care staff. Working with all of his program administrators, he was able to develop five categories of options for funding cutbacks beginning with some administrative and overhead cuts and ending with actually terminating some hospital and community services. This series of options served to educate the executive and legislative branches about what their fiscal decisions would actually mean to patients, programs, and citizens. The commissioner, further, made it clear to all concerned that he was a patient-care and program advocate and that cutting services would be the public policy decision of the governor and legislature and not his decision. He viewed it as his role to strongly educate the decision-makers and the public about the consequences of their fiscal actions.[4] The commissioner used the newspapers, radio, and television to carry his message, and the public become more knowledgeable about mental health and retardation. The superintendents and staffs of some of the facilities helped greatly in bringing our message to public and governmental attention. The governor had fortunately made this area one of the highest priorities of his administration but needed professional input about the impact of the budget on services. The state had also made a commitment to participate in the Title XIX (Medicaid) program for mental retardation and had entered into at least one consent decree to upgrade services at a state school and was soon to enter into others. Employees and citizens were also vocal about the needs of our patients.

There emerged a relatively powerful advocacy coalition of mental health and retardation groups which had previously had little in the way of working relationships. This included professional societies in psychiatry, psychology, nursing, and social work. In addition, there were self-help and advocacy groups and statewide citizen groups, such as the Mental Health Association and the Association for Retarded Citizens and the Governor's State Advisory Committee (a largely citizen group representing local mental health area boards, regional councils, and some professional interests). This Coalition for Mental Health and Retardation had a strong citizen leader and provided vigorous advocacy and support to the commissioner and the Department of Mental Health.

The commissioner was somewhat vulnerable in that his department had little accurate data documenting its services and needs. He began an office for information systems, evaluation and planning to generate basic data. He also moved to increase revenues to offset expenses and demonstrate a reduction of net cost to the state. Especially in mental retardation this was successful and revenues have increased from $24 million in 1975 to $56 million in 1978.

Furthermore, the commissioner used the crisis to close one

state hospital (long in the talking stage), consolidate hospital services, and develop community alternatives for these patients as well as new programs for children. The closing actually enhanced patient care as well as administration.[5] Planning for the closing of another hospital was also undertaken. The governor and legislature allowed the department to use savings from hospital closings for new community programs. The governor later went further with the next and permanent commissioner (Robert L. Okin, M.D., a psychiatrist) to publically state that dollars from closing state hospitals and schools would be used dollar-for-dollar for new community programs. The commissioner (LBM) also attempted to obtain more fiscal flexibility to move funds, contract for services and reallocate resources. But this will be a long time coming in our state. There was strong clarification (which the governor and legislature began to understand) of the clinical and program needs especially for both hospital and community services and not one or the other.[4]

The outcome of the 1975 crisis was that the budget, as finally passed, had some cuts in administration but not in patient care, and it totaled $198 million or close to the department's request. A modest increase in taxes also finally passed. Further, while flexibility was not obtained there have been fewer devastating hiring freezes and the decision-makers within government, as well as the public were much more knowledgeable about and sympathetic to mental health and retardation interests. Our image had greatly improved, morale had begun to redevelop and we had survived. More than that, however, we had maintained the commitment of the state to Title XIX in mental retardation, used the opportunity to begin to close more hospitals while developing high quality community care, obtained commitment from the governor (even during a fiscal crisis) and had helped to develop a new advocacy coalition of citizens and professionals.

In 1976, again under the leadership of a psychiatrist commissioner, the mental health and retardation budget grew to

$208 million, and in 1977 to $232 million primarily with increases in funds for mental retardation, Title XIX compliance. Revenues also grew as previously mentioned, providing additional third party dollars (including Medicaid, which is 50 per cent federal) to offset expenses. In addition, another hospital was closed with an actual improvement in patient care and with savings able to be used for community programs. Further, the new commissioner moved to improve administration, staffing, and management.

As the budget cycle for fiscal year 1978 approached the state was once again in serious fiscal problems, partly due to cost of living and collective bargaining increases. Once again there were serious questions of cuts in the budgets of all agencies including mental health with psychiatric training, community programs, and information systems being singled out. Once again a psychiatrist commissioner took the leadership as a patient-care advocate in educating decision-makers about the consequences of budget cuts. Once again, the Coalition for Mental Health and Retardation came to his assistance. It developed a budget subcommittee chaired by the author, then president-elect of the Massachusetts Psychiatric Society, a district branch of the American Psychiatric Association. This subcommittee independently analyzed the department's budget and then strongly advocated for its needs including making public statements and meeting in plenary sessions with the governor and secretary of Administration and Finance. The governor reiterated the priority for mental health and retardation services and subsequently submitted a $243 million budget request to the legislature, including funds for psychiatric training, $8 million for new community programs and funds for an information system. Mental health was one of a handful of state agencies that was not level-funded. However, as with other agencies in state government the Department of Mental Health was asked to absorb pay raise increases. At this writing the Massachusetts House of Representatives has increased the department's allocation to $263 million to cover between 65 and 70 per cent of the pay increases plus additional moneys for the state schools for the retarded to be Title XIX-compliant and meet judicial consent decrees. The state Senate, now working on this budget, will fully fund the department's request including the pay raise at the level of $277 million. In an additional new development the governor now meets bimonthly with the secretary of Human Services, commissioner of Mental Health, chairman of the Statewide Health Coordinating Council (a citizen) and the president of the Massachusetts Psychiatric Society to discuss issues and problems.

But while we have survived and even made use of new opportunities, we have not been without adversity in Massachusetts. We still have our funding problems (especially for new community services) and we have year-to-year budget cycles and difficulties. We are still locked into an arcane civil service and line-item budget situation. We still have a large and difficult-to-manage state bureaucracy with many external constraints from the secretaries of human services and administration and finance and the legislature. We still have a highly problemmatic certificate of need program (administered by the Department of Public Health) making changes in service and new program development at times difficult and bureaucratic. We still do not pay salaries comparable with the private sector, especially to professionals. We still have too many poorly staffed and largely custodial institutions. We still do not have an adequate mix of public, private, and medical-school-based services. Local mental health programs still cannot keep a significant share of revenues they generate in order to expand services. We have made progress in contracting and purchase of services but still have major problems especially with front-end funding. We also have ongoing problems of community acceptance of the mentally ill and retarded. We still have only a rudimentary but developing information system. We still have only a small number of trained clinician-administrators. We still are devastatingly overwhelmed with paper work and crisis-oriented planning. We still have major recruitment problems;

it is especially hard to get psychiatrists to enter our public mental health programs, make themselves a career, and not leave in frustration. In brief, we have survived and even grown and developed considerably, but we have not yet overcome.

DISCUSSION

The case illustration should be considered as the attempt of one state to deal with the current climate of adversity. Most of all, it should be clear that the situation is not hopeless for hopelessness is our greatest foe. Many things can be done and with persistence there are still opportunities for us to survive and indeed to prosper somewhat.

The lessons learned from this case illustration should be examined against the backdrop of the decline of moral treatment, if we are to recognize clearly what must be done to assure our current survival. That humanistic-interpersonal treatment movement of the first three quarters of the nineteenth century declined because of a number of identifiable factors. Four major as well as associated and contributory factors can be identified with the decline of moral treatment. Curiously they are paralleled in the current era by similar sets of issues that contribute prominently to our present state of affairs.

In the 1870s there was the death of an inspired leadership group, which had not trained its successors. This was coupled with the development of a pessimistic and hopeless view of mental illness associated with the development of the scientific medicine of the day and associated with the growth of Social Darwinism and the growing attitude in the social sphere of a survival of the fittest ethos.

Beginning in the 1870s and extending through later decades, the emphasis was on cellular and brain pathology and on categorization of the forms of mental illness with a shift away from the interpersonal and humanistic understanding of the mentally ill. In the larger society, this was associated with a shift away from the earlier concern with the individual that punctuated the pre-Civil War period in American society.

An economic recession in 1876 caused clear cutbacks in hospital services at a time when utilization was increasing due to the stresses of this economic instability and also to the reform movement of middle of the nineteenth century.

In the middle and latter decades of the nineteenth century, large waves of immigrants to this country brought many new high risk people who had significant language barriers and who were very different in culture, socioeconomic status, and education from the staffs of the institutions in which moral treatment was practiced. This produced innumerable difficulties in the practice of this form of therapy, which depended heavily on human interaction between patients and staff.

Although it had occurred earlier than the final decades of decline of moral treatment, the veto by President Franklin Pierce in 1854 of the 12.5 million acre bill was a most significant event. This bill provided for a major land sale the proceeds of which would have provided federal funding for mental health services (moral treatment at that time), something that had to wait for another hundred years. The lack of this federal funding was no doubt a forerunner of and contributor to the later decline of moral treatment.

Overburdened, understaffed, underfunded, with admissions soaring, with no successors to the early leadership group, with a society whose values were shifting, it is no wonder that moral treatment declined and the care and treatment of the seriously mentally ill became consumed by a wave of pessimism. The subsequent retrenchment in the willingness to provide the means of enlightened care for the mentally ill and the low status given psychiatry continued essentially unchanged until the late 1940s. This was despite some interest in the intellectual community in psychoanalysis, some enthusiasm generated by Adolph Meyer, and a brief flurry of interest that followed World War I. It was only during and after World War II that psychiatry and concern for the mentally ill again aroused the support of the nation.

I have traced some of the parallels to our current situation elsewhere.[6] For our purposes here, the critical issues are the hopelessness that the situation in the 1870s engendered and the sense of hopelessness that many experience today and also the problem of leadership.

If we become enmeshed in a web of pessimism, hopelessness, or apathy, state services will most likely deteriorate further. Rather, at various levels of professional activities including programs, professional societies and government we must look for opportunities and capitalize on them. Rather than throw up our hands in despair we should become leading public advocates for high-quality patient care. People in the executive and legislative branches of government will still listen to us and look to us for expertise and responsible leadership. As we become increasingly more convinced patient-care advocates, we should work with a variety of other concerned professional and citizen groups who have similar interests. If this is psychopolitics, so be it! If we believe in what we have long stood for in quality patient care we cannot shrink from operating in the political arena for that is where, increasingly, decisions about our profession and our patients are being made. This is true locally and at the state level as well as nationally as it is clear that a new initiative is essential. Politics is not a hostile arena nor are the media necessarily hostile. We must come to know these areas and their ways and work with them if we are to survive. Many of the public, their representatives, and the press want to understand us and help; it is our job to make that possible. At the same time that we are leaders in this area, we must also be collaborators. New partnerships with psychology, social work, nursing, and the paraprofessionals must emerge. We must work actively with citizen groups at national, state, and local levels. For psychiatry this means a new adjustment to a situation where we can lead but also acknowledge our shortcomings and need for collaborative assistance from others. The marriage of psychiatry with the other medical and mental health disciplines and with citizen groups is a potent political force and one that works.

Further, we must train and support a larger and growing cadre of clinician-administrators from amongst our ranks who can develop and operate programs and who are skilled in the sphere of politics. We can no longer rely on our clinical experience or scientific evidence alone to win the day; we sorely need a larger and ongoing leadership group to carry our efforts further. We cannot be blind, as were the leaders of moral treatment, to the grave need to train our successors so that what we have and will achieve can continue.

CONCLUSIONS

History teaches us many lessons about the evolution of mental health services. We can learn much from the periods of decline and our situation currently parallels one of those other decline eras.[6] We have presented a case illustration of one state's attempts to cope with this situation and have extracted from it some lessons regarding leadership, collaboration, political activity, patient advocacy, and hope. We cannot end without some cautionary questions: Can large state mental health bureaucracies really be effective? Will psychiatrists be interested and concerned with public service? Can we really develop a leadership group of clinician-administrators who are patient-care advocates and can we train our successors? Can we and do we want to endure the frustrations of public service in order to be public servants? Can states recognize that public psychiatry must be as attractive as private practice if it is to recruit well-trained professionals? Can we stand by and allow the destruction of state mental health programs?

If we can answer any of these questions in the affirmative, then hope springs eternal.

REFERENCES

1. Bennis, W. G.: "A funny thing happened on the way to the future," in *Psychology and the Problems of Society,* Korten, F., Cook, S., & Lacey, J., eds. Washington, D.C.: American Psychology Inc, 1970.

2. Macht, L. B., & Scherl, D. J.: "Facing the Nation: Some Issues and Answers for Neighborhood Psychiatry," in *Neighborhood Psychiatry,* Macht, L. B., Scherl, D. J., & Sharfstein, S., eds. Lexington, Mass.: Heath, 1977.

3. Levinson, D. J., & Klerman, G. L.: "The clinician executive." *Psychiatry* 30:1, February 1967.

4. Macht, L. B.: "Reflections on the psychiatrist as commissioner: A special case of the clinician executive." *Psychiatric Opinion,* (Accepted for publication).

5. Macht, L. B.: "The Closing of a State Mental Hospital," (In preparation).

6. Macht, L. B. Material prepared for: "The Former Mental Hospital Patient in the Community, A Report of the Group for the Advancement of Psychiatry," (In preparation).

INDEX